EAT *to* BEAT

PROSTATE CANCER
COOKBOOK

EAT *to* BEAT
PROSTATE CANCER *COOKBOOK*

by DAVID RICKETTS

FOREWORD BY SIMON J. HALL, M.D.
Director, Barbara & Maurice Deane Prostate Health & Research Center
Mount Sinai School of Medicine, New York

INTRODUCTION BY ALAN R. KRISTAL, Dr. P.H.
Associate Head, Cancer Prevention Program
Fred Hutchinson Cancer Research Center
Seattle, Washington

STEWART, TABORI & CHANG   NEW YORK

Published in 2006 by Stewart, Tabori & Chang
An imprint of Harry N. Abrams, Inc.

Library of Congress Cataloging-in-Publication Data

Ricketts, David.
  Eat to beat prostate cancer cookbook / author, David Ricketts ; foreword,
Simon J Hall; introduction, Alan R Kristal.
      p. cm.
  Includes bibliographical references and index.
  ISBN 1-58479-475-5
  1. Prostate—Cancer—Diet therapy—Recipes. I. Title.
  RC280.P7R53 2006
  641.5'631—dc22

                        2005034437

The text of this book was composed in Bembo and Trade Gothic.

DESIGNER: HOWARD KLEIN
PRODUCTION MANAGER: KIM TYNER

Printed and bound in the United States
10 9 8 7 6 5 4 3 2 1

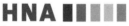

harry n. abrams, inc.
a subsidiary of La Martinière Groupe
115 West 18th Street
New York, NY 10011
www.hnabooks.com

DISCLAIMER

This book is not intended as a substitute for the medical advice of physicians. The reader should regularly consult a physician in all matters relating to his or her health, and particularly in respect of any symptoms that may require diagnosis or treatment. Neither the author nor the publisher shall be liable or responsible for any loss, injury, or damage allegedly arising from any information or suggestion in this book.

CONTENTS

PROSTATE CANCER *and* THE NEWLY DIAGNOSED: The Role of Patient and Doctor

BY SIMON J. HALL, MD

WHILE PROSTATE CANCER REMAINS THE MOST commonly diagnosed non–skin cancer in America, accounting for over 230,000 new cases in 2005, the initial diagnosis for the individual man is a disturbingly personal experience, associated with feelings of vulnerability, fear, and loneliness. For many men, this is the first time that their own mortality has come into view. In my experience, most patients are overwhelmed with these feelings of being alone, and they want to retreat and face their disease in private, even though friends and family may offer support. While dealing with these psychological issues, newly diagnosed patients at the same time must wrestle with the often difficult decision as to what is the best treatment: watchful waiting, radical prostatectomy, or the latest advances in radiation therapy and seed implantation.

At this juncture, what can a man newly diagnosed with prostate cancer do? First, it is important to understand that he is not alone. Following the diagnosis, many patients suddenly realize that they know a close friend or a distant relative who is a prostate cancer survivor. Discussions with fellow patients, whether one-on-one or through support groups, are important resources of solace, support, and information. The key issue is to communicate—and not to be afraid to talk about the disease and one's own fears.

Secondly, access to information is critically important as a man works to make his own individual choices for treatment. The more information that is available and searched out and studied, the more likely he is to be comfortable with his final treatment decision. Key to this process is a thorough self-education through books and the Internet. Equally important are consultations with a wide range of doctors, including at the very least, a urologic oncologist skilled in prostate surgery and a radiation oncologist specializing in either external beam radiation therapy or seed implantations. Many institutions now offer multidisciplinary programs where a patient and his family or support group can meet with a radiation oncologist, a urologist, and for more advanced cases, a medical oncologist, to fully discuss the patient's options, the pros and cons of each treatment, and the effects on the quality of life—and all this very often in the same session. This multidisciplinary approach can help to make these difficult decisions a little easier, although at the time it is a lot of information to absorb.

Technology, with the development by some medical institutions of computer-based interactive educational tools, can also play an important role in making the treatment decision. The use of these computer tools is not intended to make the decision for a patient, but rather to provide another source of information that will help a man to be more comfortable and more positive with his final choice. It is important to remember, that while a man is facing this potentially life-threatening disease, the vast majority of men are able to fight it on numerous levels, with an excellent chance for survival.

Sometimes, however, access to information is difficult. Many men live in areas where it is not possible to find experienced prostate cancer doctors who will talk with them about what their diagnosis means and explain all the treatment options. This dialogue becomes even more important if the initial treatment fails. For some men, it is possible to travel to a cancer center for information gathering. But for others, it's not, which further underscores the need for the patient to continually educate himself, using all the tools available, wherever he lives.

An important responsibility for the physician caring for the prostate cancer patient is to encourage him to be a more active participant in his own treatment. Many patients feel that they are at the "mercy" of physicians, and they are willing to defer to the experts. It is critically important to turn the tables so that the individual patient plays a more active role.

Since we all control what we eat, taking a look at nutrition is an excellent starting point for engaging positive feelings and proactive behavior toward one's cancer. It is clear that what we eat can significantly influence our health. And an understanding of the role of nutrition and how it can impact prostate cancer risk factors, in both a positive and a negative manner, is important for men who are concerned about their own chances of developing prostate cancer and also for those already diagnosed.

The interplay of diet and risk factors is complex. In the United States, African American men have the highest incidence of prostate cancer, while Asian men, those from

China and Japan, have the lowest. Interestingly, the autopsy examination of prostate tissues of men from different ethnic backgrounds who die without evidence of clinical prostate cancer reveals similar incidences of small, well-differentiated, latent cancers. It is thought that one of the main causes for the conversion of a latent cancer into a clinically significant cancer is the interaction between environmental factors and genetic predilection. Recent studies demonstrating the high incidence of prostate cancer in the Caribbean and West Africa suggest that men with a significant African genetic background have a higher risk and predilection for developing prostate cancer. Ongoing studies are exploring environmental factors, such as nutrition, as a way to further modify this higher risk. When Asian families emigrate to the United States, within one generation the incidence of prostate cancer rises to levels significantly higher than in China or Japan, but not to the levels of that for Caucasians and African Americans. It is unclear whether this change is due to the protective effects of the Asian diet, which is generally centered on vegetables, grains, fish, soy-based products, and teas, or the deleterious effects of the American diet, characterized by a high intake of animal-based products and a low intake of fruits and vegetables. Evidence exists supporting both theories. In either instance, it is thought that diet may help control the potential conversion of a latent cancer to a clinical cancer. Clearly, the average American eats far too much meat and associated fats and does not consume enough vegetables and fruits. Avoidance of animal fats appears to reduce the risk of developing prostate cancer as well as colon cancer and is also important for maintaining cardiovascular health. Other dietary studies, including animal studies, have explored soy and soy products, and have demonstrated that some compounds in soy have anticancer properties.

Dietary lifestyle changes require commitment and patience. Many patients, early in their diagnosis, make substantial changes in their eating routines, only to retreat to former patterns within a year. The deleterious effect of what we eat may not be years in the making, but the benefits of healthy eating, whether to prevent or treat an existing cancer, require almost daily adherence and can only be achieved through a commitment to a new lifestyle.

Another factor to consider is that food supplements, especially at higher doses, may not be harmless. In an attempt to enhance their cancer defenses, people often megadose on supplements. Many patients are familiar with the study which explored the ability of vitamin E versus a placebo to prevent lung cancer in smokers. The study noted no difference between either agent to prevent lung cancer, but it did reveal a decreased incidence of prostate cancer in the men who took vitamin E. However, what most people don't realize is that a third arm of the study demonstrated that beta-carotene actually increased the risk of lung cancer over the placebo. This shows that in many instances we clearly don't know whether we are helping or harming a patient by recommending food supplements for cancer prevention or treatment. Likewise, it is important to realize that the Food and Drug Administration has no jurisdiction over food supplements, so it is critical to purchase supplements from reliable sources—and only after you've done the research. What a label says and what in fact is in the bottle may be two different things.

While it is clear that mainstream medicine has not adequately explored the role of nutrition and food supplements in the prevention or treatment of prostate cancer, the literature is rich with numerous studies with which a patient should become familiar, either on his own or through consultation with a physician during the treatment-decision process or an ongoing follow-up. It is always important to become educated about the facts and myths, especially with regard to food supplements, such as vitamins. And be aware that many studies focus on the potential for preventing prostate cancer, which doesn't necessarily translate into helpful information for the man already diagnosed.

My essential message is that a man who is concerned about prostate cancer, whether diagnosed or not, needs to become as educated as he can about what he eats and how he supplements his dietary intake. Keep in mind that natural food sources are generally preferable to megadoses of vitamins and other supplements.

The focus of this cookbook is to present a collection of prostate-healthy recipes that will help a man to incorporate healthy eating for himself and his family and friends into his everyday life. This is a major step in the overall strategy of taking control and battling prostate cancer.

Simon J. Hall, MD, is chairman of the Department of Urology, associate professor in the Departments of Urology and Gene & Cell Medicine, and director of the Barbara & Maurice Deane Prostate Health & Research Center at the Mount Sinai School of Medicine in New York City.

Dr. Hall earned his medical degree from the College of Physicians & Surgeons, Columbia University, before receiving training at the Department of Surgery, Mount Sinai School of Medicine, and Department of Urology, Boston University Medical Center, and was subsequently awarded a two-year Uro-Oncology Fellowship, Scott Department of Urology, Baylor College of Medicine.

His research interests include the development of gene therapy strategies for the treatment of prostate cancer. Dr. Hall has received the Dr. Solomon Silver Award in Clinical Medicine, Mount Sinai School of Medicine; the Edwin Beer Award in Urology, New York Academy of Medicine; and the F. Brantly Scott Award, Scott Department of Urology, Baylor College of Medicine. Author of numerous papers on gene therapy, Dr. Hall is a section editor of gene therapy/immunotherapy, *Urologic Oncology*, serves on the examination committees of the American Board of Urology and American Urological Association, and serves as reviewer and consultant for other scientific journals.

DIET *and* DIETARY SUPPLEMENTS *and* THE PROSTATE CANCER RISK:
What the studies tell us

BY ALAN R. KRISTAL, DR. PH

MOST MEN ARE CONCERNED ABOUT prostate cancer, and they should be, especially those over forty, since prostate cancer is a relatively common disease. About one in six American men develop it. But the good news is that few men actually die of prostate cancer. This is because about 80 percent of men diagnosed with prostate cancer have disease that is localized within the prostate, and almost all of these men have a very high rate of long-term survival. Given these facts, an important question is: Are there steps a man can take to impact prostate cancer, before or after diagnosis? This is an especially important consideration for the nearly quarter million men who each year are diagnosed with prostate cancer.

One question many men ask me is whether changes in their diet or the use of dietary supplements can lower their risk of developing prostate cancer or lower the risk of their cancer recurring if they have been already diagnosed and treated. To answer this, large studies are now underway to examine the role of diet and dietary supplements in both preventing prostate cancer and lessening the chance of recurrence. But for the moment, our current base of scientific knowledge is quite limited. While waiting for the results of these studies, which will continue through the end of the decade, we can make reasonable recommendations about diet, based on two factors: our understanding of the basic molecular events that cause healthy cells to develop into cancer; and scientific studies that have examined prostate cancer in large samples of men.

What causes prostate cancer, and how can diet play a role?

Prostate cancer occurs when a group of previously healthy cells begin to grow abnormally, and as a result, change the normal architecture of the prostate gland. As mentioned above, prostate cancer is very common, and by age seventy, almost all men have small areas of cancer in their prostate. For reasons we do not understand, some of these cancers may grow into the tissue surrounding the prostate and eventually spread or metastasize into distant parts of the body. The only factors we know with some certainty to increase the risk of prostate cancer are age, the presence of a chronic inflammatory condition called prostatitis, being an African American, and having a family history of prostate cancer.

To better understand the mechanics of how cancer develops, it's useful to look at what happens on a cellular level. When a cell's DNA (the genetic code that determines cell function) is damaged (for whatever reason), the cell may begin to grow abnormally. Most of the time, damaged cells either repair their DNA or they die, thus eliminating any potential problem. But, if cells with damaged DNA survive, they can grow faster than the surrounding healthy cells. Over many years, these cells can accumulate additional DNA damage, which may cause them to develop into cancers.

Scientists believe there are two ways that DNA can be damaged: through oxidative damage caused by free radicals, and cumulative DNA damage caused by abnormally rapid cell growth.

Since diet is known to play an important role in both protecting cells from DNA damage and regulating cell growth, it's only logical to conclude that diet can also play an important role in promoting good prostate health.

Diet and Oxidative DNA Damage

Free radicals are molecules abundantly produced as a by-product of normal cellular functions or oxidation. The trouble starts when they bind directly to the DNA in a cell and damage it. But cells are not helpless. They can battle the free radicals and limit damage through two defenses: reliance on antioxidants, and their own antioxidant enzyme systems.

Many foods, in particular fruits and vegetables, contain compounds that function as antioxidants. These antioxidant compounds bind to free radicals and detoxify them before they can damage the DNA. Perhaps the best-known dietary antioxidants are vitamins E and C, but there are thousands of others that are believed to be effective, especially when several work together. This large group of antioxidants includes carotenoids (the dark pigments found in tomatoes, carrots, and many other plant foods) and the phenols and flavonoids (responsible for the pungent flavors in some fruits, vegetables, and herbs). In contrast, some foods, such as grilled meats and polyunsaturated oils, may, in fact, increase the levels of free radicals and promote DNA damage.

A cell's own antioxidant enzyme systems can also detoxify free radicals by converting them into inert compounds that are excreted from the cell. To function effectively, some of these enzyme systems require specific nutrients, such as selenium or zinc. Other systems are stimulated by certain compounds in particular foods, such as broccoli and cabbage, which are members of the cruciferous family of vegetables.

Diet and Cell Growth

Prostate cell growth is mainly affected by three important determinants. The first involves male (androgen) and female (estrogen) steroid hormones, both of which men produce. As men age, their androgen activity decreases, while their estrogen activity stays relatively constant, although it may drop and then plateau. These two factors usually translate into slower prostate cell growth. But high-energy (calorie), high-fat, low-fiber dietary patterns, as well as obesity, can increase levels of steroid hormones in the blood, and this in turn can stimulate prostate cell growth, even in aging men.

The metabolism of steroid hormones can also be affected by particular dietary compounds, causing the hormones to become more or less biologically active. For example, compounds found in Brussels sprouts cause estrogens to metabolize into biologically inactive compounds.

Inflammation is the second important determinant in prostate cell growth. It's the response to an infection or other types of tissue injury, which causes cells to die, and in turn, stimulates new cells to grow as replacements. The severe, chronic inflammation tied to prostate cancer, called prostatitis, is relatively rare, but it can cause cell growth. More commonly found in otherwise healthy prostate tissue during microscopic examination are small, multiple areas of chronic inflammation. Recent studies suggest that these small areas may be the earliest detectable changes in cells that are on their way to becoming cancer.

How does diet relate to inflammation? The fats known as omega-3s that are found in fish can profoundly reduce the inflammatory response in cells. In contrast, the trans fats found in some snack chips and vegetable oils can promote inflammation. But more about this later.

The third growth determinant involves many molecules that are called "growth factors" and they determine how cells develop. In some foods there is a class of growth factors, such as vitamins D and A, that cause cells to normally mature and then naturally lose their reproductive potential—that's a good thing. Other growth factors are produced in response to certain compounds in foods, and this can be a bad thing. For example, the "insulin-like growth factor type 1," or IGF-1, is associated with both prostate cell growth and an increased risk of prostate cancer, and the amount of it found in the blood is increased by diets high in protein and milk.

Avoid

Based on studies, which dietary patterns, foods, or nutrients can reduce prostate cancer risk?

A diet that lowers prostate cancer risk generally:

> provides antioxidants and stimulates antioxidant enzyme systems

> reduces androgens and androgen activity

> reduces inflammation

> reduces or controls growth factors that cause cells to rapidly grow

Let's consider each of these characteristics in turn.

Provides antioxidants and stimulates antioxidant enzyme systems

Antioxidants and pro-oxidants. Many studies have tied antioxidants to a lower risk of prostate cancer, but the story is not altogether clear. Generally, it is thought that vegetables, which contain a wide variety of antioxidants, are associated with a lower risk of prostate cancer, and that seems to be underscored by several studies. However, the evidence that any specific antioxidant is responsible for this lowering of risk is more limited. For example, the evidence for lycopene (the red pigment in tomatoes and watermelon), is based primarily on only one large study, which found that men who ate dishes made with tomato sauce, such as pizza and pasta, had a 16 percent lower risk of prostate cancer.

Evidence for resveritrol (a flavonoid in red wine and red grapes) reducing prostate cancer risk is also from a single study, which concluded that a daily glass of red wine (but not white wine or other alcoholic beverages) decreased risk by 6 percent.

The best evidence for any particular antioxidant is for vitamin E, especially among smokers. A large study evaluating whether vitamin E could prevent lung cancer in smokers found that the vitamin had no effect on lung cancer, but that it did lower the risk of prostate cancer in these men by 32 percent. Perhaps men exposed to high levels of environmental toxins, such as cigarette smoke, need the extra antioxidant protection provided by vitamin E.

A large trial, called the Selenium and Vitamin E Cancer Prevention Trial (SELECT), is currently underway, testing whether vitamin E supplements (400 mg/day) can reduce prostate cancer risk. But the results will not be available until at least 2010.

Other studies have clearly indicated that vitamin C, whether in foods, multivitamins, or high-dose supplements, is *not* associated with prostate cancer, although it does have strong antioxidant properties.

And while there are many studies examining the effects of antioxidant compounds on cancer cells grown in test-tube cultures, it is highly unlikely that many of these experiments in test tubes will tell us much about what these antioxidants will do in humans.

In addition to antioxidants, some foods contain pro-oxidants, which have been associated with increased prostate cancer risk. One of the chief offenders in this category is red meat, which in some studies has been associated with increased risk. The reason for this may be that grilling or frying meats produces compounds that act like very potent free radicals.

Antioxidant enzyme systems. In contrast to the unclear evidence about any specific antioxidant, some foods and nutrients affecting antioxidant enzyme systems have been consistently associated with reduced prostate cancer risk.

Selenium, which is a key component of several antioxidant enzymes, has been strongly associated with reduced prostate cancer risk across many studies. The same large trial (SELECT) testing vitamin E is also testing selenium supplementation, so a more definitive answer will be available at the end of the decade. Selenium is found in many foods, including whole grains, seafood, and garlic. For plant sources of selenium, the concentration depends upon where the food is grown. The soil in some parts of the U.S., particularly the Southeast, is low in selenium, and men living in these states may have low selenium intakes.

Cruciferous vegetables, which include broccoli, Brussels sprouts, cabbage, mustard greens, and bok choy, contain compounds that both increase the activity of certain antioxidant enzymes and lower the activity of some steroid hormones. These vegetables have been consistently associated with lower overall cancer risk, and there is growing evidence for their effect on prostate cancer as well. Here's a tip: You get the most benefit from cruciferous vegetables when you eat them raw. This is because the compounds responsible for their biological activity, called isothiocyanates, are formed when an enzyme in the plant cell wall is released by chewing. Cooking completely inactivates this enzyme. Eating broccoli sprouts or raw broccoli in salads is the best way to maximize the benefit from cruciferous vegetables.

Reduces androgens and androgen activity

Many studies have found that a "Western" dietary pattern—high in energy (calorie) and saturated fat and low in fiber—is associated with increased androgen and estrogen activity, and consequently, presents a higher risk of prostate cancer. Saturated fats are found in meats and full-fat dairy products, and fiber is found in fruits, vegetables, and whole-grain foods. There is some evidence that diets high in saturated fat may increase the risk of dying from prostate cancer once diagnosed.

Obesity is also associated with steroid hormones, although the associations of obesity with prostate cancer are complex. Obesity does not appear to increase the risk of getting prostate cancer, but it does seem to increase the risk of dying from it once you have it. Obesity and high-fat dietary patterns are strongly linked, especially in the United States and other industrialized countries, and together they seem to increase the risk of heart disease and many cancers, including prostate cancer.

Reduces inflammation

The most familiar way to reduce inflammation, which can lead to increased cell growth, is with over-the-counter drugs such as aspirin and ibuprofen. Several studies have found that long-term, high-dose aspirin use decreases prostate cancer risk, but at the same time, the side effects of aspirin (as well as other nonsteroidal inflammatory drugs) may cause significant harm.

Here diet enters the picture again. As I mentioned before, the omega-3 polyunsaturated fats found in fish, in particular oily or dark fish such as salmon and mackerel, are also strong anti-inflammatory agents, and fish consumption appears to be free of harmful side effects (although there is increasing discussion about the levels of PCBs and mercury in fish; see page 189). Studies are not altogether consistent, but several do find that men who eat fish regularly are at lower risk for prostate cancer.

In contrast, another group of fats, called trans fats, has strong pro-inflammatory effects. Trans fats are formed when fats are processed (hydrogenated) in order to promote a long shelf life, and they are often used in margarine, cookies, crackers, snack chips, and in frying fat used by fast-food restaurants. Multiple studies have found that trans fats increase the risk of heart disease, and recent studies are finding that they may increase the risk of prostate cancer as well. Trans fats can easily be avoided, since new food labeling regulations require information about trans fat content. And many food manufacturers are reformulating their foods to eliminate trans fats.

Reduces or controls growth factors that cause cells to rapidly grow

This is one of the more controversial and uncertain areas of research in diet and prostate cancer. It is clear from animal studies that insulin and the insulinlike growth factors play an important role in prostate cell growth and perhaps in cancer generally. Obesity significantly increases insulin levels, as does eating foods with sugars (carbohydrates) that are rapidly absorbed into the bloodstream. These foods, termed high-glycemic-index foods because they cause a rapid rise in blood glucose, include sweetened carbonated beverages, candy, breads, sweetened cereals made with processed grains rather than whole grains, and even potatoes. But the evidence is scant that these foods may actually increase prostate cancer risk.

Generally, the dietary factors that increase insulinlike growth factors are high total energy or caloric intake, excessive protein (especially animal protein), and excessive milk consumption. Low-energy diets are consistently associated with lower cancer risk, including prostate cancer. Although studies generally find no association between protein and prostate cancer, many find that dairy foods, especially milk, do increase prostate cancer risk. And to confuse matters even more, there are parallel findings for calcium, whether consumed from foods or supplements. Dairy foods contain growth factors that have been secreted into milk, and perhaps these affect prostate cell growth. Dairy foods also contain large amounts of calcium, and due to a complex system regulating bone health, high dietary calcium intake lowers serum levels of vitamin D. Since vitamin D acts as the opposite of a growth factor, lower levels may lead to higher rates of cell growth. Calcium is an important nutrient for bone health, and it lowers colon cancer risk. Careful moderation of calcium is needed to balance its beneficial and potentially harmful effects.

There are some compounds in foods that can also affect the complex signaling pathways that ultimately cause cells to replicate. For example, in cell culture studies it has been shown that genistein (an isoflavone) in soy foods, catechines in green tea, and limonene from citrus fruit peel, all interfere with signaling pathways, causing cells with damaged DNA to die instead of replicating. There are a few studies that have found that men who eat soy foods have lower prostate cancer risk, but the evidence is not strong. Since few men in this country drink green tea, eat soy foods, or consume large amounts of citrus peel, it is difficult to evaluate the effects of these compounds, even in retrospective studies. Some scientists have questioned the safety of eating large amounts of soy foods because some compounds in soy can also function as very weak estrogens, causing cell growth.

Recommendations and guidelines

Given all the uncertainty as I've outlined above, what recommendations make the most sense? There are several recurrent themes in studies relating diet to prostate cancer risk. These are:

> Maintain a healthy weight. Balance calorie intake with exercise.

> Eat a variety of vegetables, both cooked and raw.

> Moderate total and saturated fat intakes.

> Moderate consumption of red meat, especially grilled and fried.

> Choose margarine, cookies, crackers, and other processed foods containing no trans fats.

> Select foods in fast-food restaurants that are not fried in oil containing trans fats.

> Eat at least one serving (and preferably more) of dark-fleshed fish per week.

> Choose breads and cereals made with whole grains.

> Moderate milk and calcium consumption.

We lack sufficient evidence to make recommendations for supplementation, either for nutrients or compounds found in herbs and other plants. If you choose to use dietary supplements, limit vitamin E to no more than 400 mg/day, selenium to no more that 200 mcg/day, and calcium to no more than 400 mg/day.

This cookbook offers practical information on how to apply these guidelines to meal planning, as well as to the selection of ingredients and their preparation. The reduced-fat recipes stress alternatives to red meat and dairy products and focus on fruits and vegetables, vegetarian main dishes, fish preparations, and the incorporation of a variety of soy products into everyday meal planning. The goal is to appeal to a broad range of food tastes and still satisfy the recommendations that I've outlined above.

Alan R. Kristal, Dr. PH, is member and associate head of the Cancer Prevention Program at the Fred Hutchinson Cancer Research Center in Seattle, Washington, and professor in the Department of Epidemiology and Nutritional Sciences Program, University of Washington, Seattle.

Dr. Kristal earned his MS from Framingham State College, his MPH from Northwestern University, and Dr. PH from Columbia University. His primary research interests are in nutritional epidemiology, including the etiologic relationships between diet and cancer and implementation and evaluation of public health nutrition interventions. His current projects include studies on the interrelationships of diet, steroid hormones, growth factors, inflammation, oxidative stress, and prostate cancer risk; steroid hormones, diet, and obesity and risk of symptomatic benign prostatic hyperplasia (BPH); diet and obesity and the progression of Barrett's esophagus to esophageal adenocarcinoma; and diet and obesity and the risks of pancreas cancer.

He is also a senior editor of *Cancer Epidemiology, Biomarkers & Prevention* and associate editor of the *American Journal of Epidemiology*.

CHAPTER I

PROSTATE-HEALTHY EATING

My Diagnosis and Diet

Eat to Beat Prostate Cancer is a collection of prostate-healthy recipes that I have been developing with friends, coworkers, and health professionals during the past several years. The food reflects the way I've been eating since I was diagnosed with prostate cancer in April 2001 at age fifty-five. Very early in my treatment, one of my doctors strongly suggested that I tackle a low-calorie, low-fat, high-fiber, no-red-meat diet, with fish two or three times a week, grains and beans, lots of fruits and vegetables, and soy products. Since I've been a cookbook author and food writer for many years, eating good food was, and still is, high on my list of priorities. I accepted the doctor's suggestion as a culinary challenge. What did I have to lose—it was my life.

Initially, a PSA of 32 prompted me to have a prostate biopsy, which confirmed the diagnosis, with a Gleason Score of 6. (Until recently a PSA of 4.0 or less was thought to be "normal"—many doctors now suggest lowering that standard to 1.5.) In August 2001, I had a radical prostatectomy, my Gleason was upgraded to 7, and in January 2002, because my PSA never became undetectable, I began a seven-and-a-half-week course of external beam radiation. As I was working with my doctors to make these initial treatment decisions, it became clear to me that my diet was the one thing I could control on my own, and it was an area where I had enough expertise and experience to take a creative but sensible approach. And there was some scientific evidence that diet could make a difference. While revamping my meal planning, I began to think about developing recipes for a cookbook. As I complete this manuscript, my PSA hovers around 1, I'm healthy and active, and I've been on no other therapy since 2002, except a prostate-healthy diet.

Prior to my diagnosis, I was enjoying a reasonably healthy diet, emphasizing fruits and vegetables—but I must admit, there were the more-than-occasional cheddar-bacon burger, aged prime steak, and French-fried onion rings. And butter and cream could always be spotted on the top shelf in my refrigerator. I've changed all that now. I decided to follow the doctor's orders, and I even went one step further. I've given up all red meat, pork, and poultry—and as a result, I've eliminated practically all saturated fat and reduced my overall caloric intake. I stopped eating dairy products, since there is some evidence supporting the relationship between dairy products and increased prostate cell growth—no cheese, no milk, no sour cream, no heavy cream, and so on. Egg whites are okay, but no egg yolks. I increased the amount of fiber and antioxidants in my diet by using more vegetables and fruit, as well as beans and grains, in my meal planning. And I routinely incorporate tofu and other soy products into my cooking as sources of isoflavones and nonanimal protein. (For more about isoflavones and other prostate-protective substances found in certain foods, turn to "Primer of Good Nutrition and Healthy Prostate Eating," page 26.) My eating plan may be a little vigorous for some, but for me, it has worked on several different levels.

Within the first three months of this diet changeover, I lost about six pounds, my cholesterol dropped twenty points, and my energy levels noticeably increased. As it turns out, medical research indicates that the eating style I've adopted is not only helping to keep my cancer at bay, but it is also heart-healthy, reducing my risk of developing heart disease, high blood pressure, and diabetes. This means the recipes in *Eat to Beat Prostate Cancer* are not just for the prostate-health-attuned man, but they also offer other nutritional and health benefits for your family and friends who share your meals.

I've come to prefer my new way of eating and rarely miss the food I've given up. On occasion, I do have a chicken Caesar salad or a turkey salad sandwich, and if I'm eating in a restaurant with a friend who orders a T-bone, I'll sneak a taste. Otherwise, I stick very closely to my diet, and I haven't found it difficult at all. In fact, I ran into only one negative side effect, and that was increased intestinal gas and flatulence early on. This was only because my digestive system wasn't used to the amount of high-fiber and soy foods I was eating. It all settled down once my body made the adjustment—but be forewarned!

The Recipes

The recipes in *Eat to Beat Prostate Cancer Cookbook* reflect my personal style of eating, which includes everything from "comfort food" casseroles, sandwiches, and spaghetti and meatballs, to chocolate mousse and cheesecake. I took many of my old favorite recipes, such as franks and beans, cheese enchiladas, the classic Reuben sandwich, and beef stroganoff, and with a few twists and turns, transformed them into prostate-healthy versions. (But you can still keep meat-eating family members and friends happy by making half of a recipe with the soy alternative and half with meat.) Creating these new recipes was easy because there are so many good alternative food products available on supermarket shelves and in health food stores these days. But my food strategies didn't stop with reshaping popular American classics. I've included a wide range of favorite ethnic dishes—Mexican, Caribbean, Peruvian, Thai, Chinese, Indian, and Greek, to mention some—which frequently rely more on beans, grains, fruit, and vegetables, and less on meat and other animal products such as eggs and cheese.

I like to have several small meals during the day, heading for the kitchen when I begin to feel the first little growl of hunger. Some people call this "grazing" or "foraging," but I call it healthy eating. One of the benefits is that I find my energy level remains constant throughout the day and I don't experience those highs and lows that were so common when I was eating three squares a day. And I've discovered that eating mini meals and never letting myself get really hungry helps me resist the temptation of foods I'm not supposed to be eating, which are often high-fat snack munchies.

Although my eating strategies are perhaps a little easier for me to follow because I work at home, the same healthy eating tactics can also be applied to most office settings. You can always pack your own lunch. Good choices are a salmon salad sandwich (page 81), a tuna salad sandwich (page 82), or a ham and cheese roll-up (page 84). If there is a microwave in your office snack room, you can warm up one of the soups from the soup chapter. And many of the snacks and legume and grain salads from the salad chapter are easily transportable. If you're adventuresome, explore the neighborhood around your office to become familiar with health food stores, delis, and restaurants that offer prostate-healthy takeout— you will be surprised what you can find.

Even though I'm a single sixty-year-old male, I still cook for a lot of other people. Some of my recipe tasters include a middle-aged housewife who has to get dinner on the table for her family, other prostate cancer survivors, a single male who has no idea how to cook, a six-year-old girl and her friends, a professional food stylist, my ninety-year-old parents, and a registered dietician. Their responses were often eye-opening. When I passed around samples of my Spicy Cabbage Salad with Cider Vinegar (page 120), the food stylist thought it much too hot, while the six-year-old and the single male who doesn't cook loved it.

As I developed my recipes, an experienced nutritionist analyzed each one to keep track of calories, overall fat as well as saturated fat, protein, carbohydrate, fiber, sodium, and cholesterol. And a registered dietician helped me with some of the recipe development as well as answering my questions about nutrition.

Since all the recipes are generally low-calorie and low-fat, I decided not to include a nutrition analysis for each recipe. However, I do point out specific recipes that are nutritionally noteworthy—such as those that are particularly high-fiber or with no fat.

Whoever's doing the cooking in your house—you, your wife, or a significant other—they will find that the food in this cookbook is not only quite tasty and nutritious, but that it is also easy to make.

As a footnote, it is useful to mention that many of the recipes can be "beefed up" to satisfy the meat cravings of family members and friends. For instance, ground beef can be added to the Mexican Corn Stew with Red Beans and Chiles (page 104), shredded cooked chicken to the Red Rice Salad with Lime-Mustard Dressing (page 132), and small pieces of cooked meat to most of the grain and legume recipes in the Vegetarian Main Dishes chapter.

Significant Statistics

Without a lot of fanfare, prostate cancer has become a major disease. It's the number-one non–skin cancer in the United States and the third most common cancer worldwide. Almost two million men in the United States have prostate cancer, with an estimated 232,000 new cases diagnosed each year. More than thirty thousand men die each year of the disease (that's about eighty-two a day), making it the second leading cause of cancer death for men, after lung cancer. These are significant statistics. The good news is that prostate cancer is a slow grower.

For many years, there was little talk about prostate cancer, for two basic reasons: Many men went undiagnosed because of inadequate screening, and if diagnosed, they were too embarrassed to make even a passing reference to the disease because of some of the potential treatment side effects, impotence and incontinence. However, this hiding in the shadows has begun to change. Count on the glare of celebrity status to make the public more aware, as more and more prominent men are diagnosed—presidential hopeful Senator John Kerry, Secretary of State Colin Powell, ex-mayor of New York City Rudy Giuliani, evangelist Pat Robertson, actor Robert DeNiro, baseball manager Joe Torre, singer Harry Belafonte, University of Connecticut basketball coach Jim Calhoun, Emperor Akihito of Japan, and the original Viagra poster boy, former senator and presidential candidate Bob Dole.

Taking Control

A diagnosis of prostate cancer knocks the wind out of a man, since it's a disease that profoundly affects his life, striking at the core of his sexual identity. The initial assessment of how far the disease has progressed is often difficult, and the treatment options can be overwhelming. Dr. Simon J. Hall writes about how these uncertainties can affect the newly diagnosed in the Foreword (page 9).

As I was dealing with my own diagnosis as a "newbie" and trying to become comfortable with the fact that I was now a member of a special club called the "reluctant brotherhood," I explored as much material as I could about the disease wherever I could find it. I read books; checked out relevant Web sites and joined online chat groups; participated in support groups; and spoke with a range of doctors, as well as other newly diagnosed men and men who were prostate cancer survivors. I soon began to realize that an important part of my treatment should focus on what I was eating, and that was something I could immediately get a grip on.

An increasing number of studies and clinical trials underscore the relationship between diet and diet supplements and prostate cancer, lending further support to my dietary approach. Epidemiologist Dr. Alan R. Kristal reviews the highlights of all this work and makes some general dietary recommendations in the Introduction (page 13).

Exercise is also important in the fight against prostate cancer. At the time of my diagnosis, I was fifty-five and already engaged in an exercise program that included jogging, light weight lifting, and yoga. I've continued with this exercise regimen, and recent research linking the positive effects of exercise with inhibiting the development of advanced prostate cancer indicates that I've been on the right track.

Since prostate cancer has slowly come out of the closet, more men are being diagnosed earlier, and many are living for decades after diagnosis, usually in excellent health despite the cancer. That's why, for these men especially, living a healthy lifestyle that includes eating well and getting regular exercise is becoming increasingly important.

Primer of Good Nutrition and Prostate-Healthy Eating

The recipes in *Eat to Beat Prostate Cancer Cookbook* are part of my eating routine, which is generally low-calorie, low-fat (and especially low-saturated-fat), dairy-free, high-fiber, and antioxidant-rich, and includes moderate amounts of soy. These are the choices that I've made, but they may not be appropriate for everyone. However, in order to ensure a general understanding of the connection between diet and prostate-healthy eating, here follows a discussion of terms, foods, nutrients, and various compounds found in foods that are referred to throughout this cookbook.

Antioxidants. These are certain vitamins and other substances in plant foods that help fight toxic substances in the body that can cause disease. In a very simple way the body acts like a car, in that it runs by taking in fuel and burning it. Toxic exhausts or substances known as free radicals are created metabolically within the body through an oxidation process. Free radicals can damage cells, especially their DNA, which can then lead to abnormal cell behavior and eventually to disease, including cancer. Antioxidants fight off the free radicals by neutralizing them and thus help to short-circuit the disease process and protect against DNA damage. Some of the most familiar antioxidants are vitamin C, vitamin E, and beta-carotene, and then there is the mineral selenium, which acts as an antioxidant. Although each antioxidant has a unique set of characteristics and functions in a particular way, chemically and biologically, there is evidence that when groups of antioxidants work synergistically, they can effectively combat disease. That is why it is so important to a have a varied and balanced diet that includes a wide range of fruits and vegetables. The USDA Food Pyramid recommends five to nine servings of fruits and vegetables a day—that's $2\frac{1}{2}$ cups of vegetables and 2 cups of fruit.

Avocado. New research indicates that nutrients in avocados may work to inhibit the growth of prostate cancer cells and perhaps even reduce the risk of prostate cancer. The natural fat in avocados, which includes a high proportion of monounsaturated fat, may help the body to better absorb carotenoids such as lycopene and lutein that act as antioxidants. Avocado is also a good source of heart-healthy, plant-derived omega-3 fatty acids, vitamin E, and fiber. A salad made with slices of avocado and orange segments and dressed with a citrus vinaigrette is an easy way to work avocados into your meal planning. For the summer months, Chilled Avocado Soup with Chiles and Lime (page 115) is a delicious meal break.

Beans. You'll find beans in almost every cuisine in the world, and there are good reasons for that. Fresh and dried shell bells are a nutritionally powerful food and a must-have in most diets for optimal health. Here's what you get from an average cup of beans:

> about 225 calories

> one third of a day's requirement for protein

> more than half the daily requirement of the B vitamin folate

> 8 to 10 grams of fiber

> the minerals iron, magnesium, phosphorus, and zinc

Nutritionists recommend getting at least 25 grams of fiber daily. Well known for the "musical effect" they sometimes have on the digestive system, beans and other high-fiber foods can upset your stomach and intestinal tract if you're not used to eating them. To avoid discomfort, slowly increase the amount of fiber you eat over a period of a couple of weeks until you reach the recommended level.

Bell pepper. One half cup of chopped bell pepper (of any color) provides more than 150 percent of the daily requirement for vitamin C, along with a substantial amount of the antioxidant beta-carotene, which helps fight chronic disease. Bell peppers belong to the capsicum family, which includes all peppers, mild or hot, and contain small amounts of capsaicin, the compound that gives peppers their spicy heat and is often used to relieve pain.

Beta-carotene. This is the pigment that makes carrots, sweet potatoes, winter squash, and other fruits and vegetables orange. It's a member of the carotenoid family, a huge group of phytochemicals, and acts as an antioxidant in the body.

Broccoli. A cruciferous vegetable, broccoli is one of the most nutritious foods you can eat. Its flowery crown, which contains more nutrients than the stem, is superhigh in the antioxidants beta-carotene and vitamin C, plus calcium, fiber, and the B vitamin folic acid. Broccoli is also loaded with sulforaphane, a phytochemical that is thought to help fight prostate cancer by increasing the number of enzymes in the body that neutralize cancer-causing chemicals or free radicals. Ironically, the sulfur compounds that make broccoli and other members of the cabbage family so healthful are the same substances that contribute to the odor and flavor that develop during cooking, which so many people find offensive. The only way to truly enjoy broccoli and its odorous and equally healthful relatives—cauliflower, cabbage, and Brussels sprouts—is to avoid overcooking. For the best advantage, eat them raw whenever possible.

Calcium. Recent work at Harvard University strongly suggests that men who exceed 1,500 mg of calcium a day may increase their risk for advanced prostate cancer. Some researchers believe that a high calcium intake lowers the levels of vitamin D in the blood, which may in turn encourage the rapid growth of damaged cells. Most experts recommend 1,200 mg a day for men. The issue becomes more complex when a man experiences bone density loss or osteoporosis and as a result needs more calcium in his diet—the balance between calcium, vitamin D, prostate cancer, and bone loss is not clearly understood.

Carotenoids. These phytochemicals function as important antioxidants and in addition create the pigments that color certain vegetables and fruits red, orange, and yellow. Intensely colored foods, such as tomatoes, pumpkin, carrots, sweet potatoes, apricots, and mangoes, are already part of most people's diets. The antioxidant beta-carotene is probably the best known phytonutrient in this group. Lycopene (see page 32) and lutein, which is present in avocado, corn, kale, and spinach, are two other well-known carotenoids.

Citrus. Oranges, lemons, limes, and other citrus fruits are loaded with vitamin C, an antioxidant that seeks out and destroys harmful compounds in the body. (Grapefruit and grapefruit juice can be tricky, since they can interfere with the absorption of some drugs. Check with your doctor about this.) Because of its antioxidant powers, vitamin C and the foods that contain it have long been touted as cancer fighters, although this vitamin's relationship to prostate cancer is somewhat controversial. It is not known whether high doses of vitamin C have a positive, negative, or neutral effect on prostate cancer cells because studies have not shown consistent results. Some medical experts who specialize in prostate cancer recommend a diet that provides up to four times the recommended dietary allowance of vitamin C, but they emphasize that all vitamin C should come from fruits and vegetables, not supplements.

Citrus pectin, a fiber found in oranges and other citrus fruits, may help prevent prostate cancer by interfering with the spread and overgrowth of cells that lead to malignancy. Experts recommend eating whole citrus fruits rather than drinking juice, because the highest concentration of pectin is in the flesh and in the membranes that separate each segment. However, since pectin is not well absorbed into the body, scientists have developed a method to break down the fiber into smaller, more digestible pieces that can then be used to make modified citrus pectin (MCP) supplements. These supplements have been used in research to slow the rate of PSA increase in men with prostate cancer who have low levels of PSA.

Cruciferous vegetables. This family of vegetables contains a variety of phytochemicals, such as indoles and sulforaphanes, that are thought to protect against prostate cancer and breast cancer and other hormone-sensitive diseases. The vegetables include cabbage, broccoli, Brussels sprouts, cauliflower, kale, mustard greens, and watercress.

Edamame. Fresh green or immature soybeans, known as edamame (pronounced ee-du-*ma*-may) have a somewhat sweet, nutty flavor and a texture similar to lima beans. They are sold fresh or frozen, both shelled and in their pods (in which case the beans must be removed like peas from their pods). The frozen shelled edamame in plastic bags have already been blanched, so they only need a few minutes of cooking time in boiling water. Soybeans are considered by some to be an essential ingredient in a diet for healthy prostate eating because the phytochemicals they contain have been shown in laboratory studies to lower PSA levels and reduce the size of tumors. Soybeans are also an excellent source of protein, without all the saturated fat that characterizes animal sources. Edamame are sometimes served as a side-dish vegetable and often eaten out of hand as a snack, like peanuts. They add a protein boost to salads, soups, and pasta dishes. Two-thirds of a cup of frozen shelled and par-cooked edamame contains 10 grams soy protein, 4 grams fiber, 5 grams fat (mainly heart-healthy polyunsaturated and monounsaturated), 120 calories, and 10 percent of the daily requirement of calcium. Look for certified organic and non–genetically modified beans. The FDA and others recommend 25 grams of soy protein a day as part of a heart-healthy eating plan.

Fats. There are three basic types of fat: saturated, polyunsaturated, and monounsaturated. Saturated fat has been linked to heart disease and a variety of other maladies, while the unsaturated fats—monounsaturated and polyunsaturated—have been connected to lower cholesterol levels and a lower risk of heart disease. The primary sources of saturated fat are whole-milk products, red meat, and coconut milk. Monounsaturated fat is found in olives and olive oil, almonds and most other nuts, and avocados, while polyunsaturated fat is mainly derived from fatty fish, and corn, soybean, and safflower oils. And then there are the trans fats, which have been linked to higher rates of heart disease, and these fats are found in most margarines, vegetable shortening, partially hydrogenated vegetable oil, and most commercially baked goods.

The links between dietary fat and prostate cancer need more study, although some maintain that the amount of dietary fat may have more of an impact on the increased risk of metastatic prostate cancer than on the increased risk of localized prostate cancer. Since animal fat is the suspected culprit, the inference is that the consumption of heart-healthy unsaturated fats will not increase the risk of prostate cancer.

Free radicals. See antioxidants.

Fiber. Fiber began to receive a lot of attention in the press a few years ago with all the hoopla about oat bran and its healthful properties. Fiber is an important element in a healthy diet, and Americans usually don't get enough of it. Fiber has been linked to cancer prevention, cholesterol reduction, and the lowering of the risk of heart disease and diabetes. And some make the argument that soluble fiber can lower the amount of testosterone in the blood, which is known to spur the growth of prostate cancer cells. Soluble fiber binds with fatty acids and digestive juices and prolongs digestive time, while insoluble fiber moves bulk through the intestines, promoting regular bowel movements. Sources of soluble fiber include oats and oat bran; nuts; dried beans (including soybeans) and peas; fruits such as oranges, apples, strawberries, blueberries, and dried fruits; and vegetables such as Brussels sprouts and carrots. Insoluble fiber is found in whole-wheat products including bulghur, barley, couscous, and brown rice; vegetables such as green beans and cauliflower; and potato and fruit skins. Current recommendations suggest that adults consume 20 to 35 grams of dietary fiber a day.

Flavonoids. This group of phytochemicals with antioxidant properties is found in broccoli, carrots, onions, soybeans, and lots of other foods. Flavonoids are the active ingredient in red wine and green tea, thought to have prostate cancer–fighting properties.

Green tea. Some recent studies have shown that a polyphenol in green tea called EGCG, an antioxidant, may prevent cancer cells from growing. Other studies have suggested that catechins and other polyphenols (flavonoids) in green tea may inhibit cancer growth in the early stages, but that catechins probably have no effect in the more advanced stages. At this point, the evidence is inconclusive as to how effective green tea polyphenols may be. However, it is known that these polyphenols are sensitive to air and light, but are more stable in the presence of acid and vitamin C—so here is another reason to squirt a little lemon in your tea.

Isoflavones. These are phytochemicals found in soybeans and other legumes, which act as antioxidants and contain biologically active plant estrogens that can mimic or inhibit the action of estrogen as a growth hormone in the body. Studies of isoflavones in laboratory animals with prostate cancer have shown a reduction of the number and size of tumors. Two isoflavones, genistein and daidzein, appear to have the most positive effect. Research also suggests that soy consumed in combination with green or black tea may have even more powerful anti–prostate cancer effects. Although genistein may help lower PSA levels, a high intake has also been shown to have adverse effects on health. Experts recommend getting your isoflavones from food sources only, especially soy food products, rather than supplements, since the soy foods eaten on any diet are unlikely to cause problems and are probably better utilized by the body.

To get more isoflavones in your diet, replace meat, poultry, dairy products, and other animal foods with tofu, soy milk, soy cheeses, soy cold cuts, and other soybean products. You'll find a wide variety of these in any health food store and in the healthy foods section of many supermarkets. Some researchers suggest 50 to 100 mg a day.

Soy Isoflavone Content*

SOY FOOD	SERVING	ISOFLAVONES (MG)
Soybeans, uncooked mature	½ cup	176 mg
Soybeans, roasted	½ cup	167 mg
Soybeans, fresh green, uncooked	½ cup	70 mg
Soy flour	¼ cup	44 mg
Tofu, uncooked	4 ounces	38 mg
Soy milk	1 cup	20 mg

*from Extension Nutrition Specialists, Cooperative Extension Service, University of Arkansas.

Lycopene. This powerful antioxidant is a carotenoid and is the pigment responsible for the red color in tomatoes, watermelon, pink grapefruit, and guava. There is strong evidence that tomatoes, and especially cooked tomato products, may reduce the risk of prostate cancer and also be particularly effective in inhibiting cancer growth in the advanced stages. Cooking tomato in a little bit of olive oil increases the body's absorption of lycopene. In addition to "An apple a day," perhaps the mantra should include "A tomato a day keeps the oncologist away."

If you start each day with an eight-ounce glass of tomato juice and work in a couple of dinners a week that include a vegetarian chili, pasta with tomato sauce, or fish with a tomato-based sauce, you're well on your way to increasing your lycopene intake naturally.

Some doctors recommend taking 30 mg of a lycopene supplement a day. Lycopene is stored in the body, so once you begin the supplement, your lycopene levels will increase and remain that way for a period of time.

Here are the amounts of lycopene in average serving sizes of popular tomato products. Keep in mind that watermelon, pink guava, pink grapefruit, and papaya are also rich sources of lycopene.

Lypocene Content

PRODUCT	SERVING SIZE	LYCOPENE (MG)
Spaghetti/marinara sauce	½ cup	20.0
Tomato sauce	½ cup	19.6
Tomato-based vegetable juice	¾ cup	17.7
Tomatoes, canned	½ cup	11.6
Tomato puree	¼ cup	10.5
Tomato paste	2 tablespoons	9.7
Tomato ketchup	2 tablespoons	5.1
Tomato, raw	1 large (about 1 cup chopped)	5.5

Olive oil. A significant portion of olive oil is heart-healthy monounsaturated fat—72 percent, in fact, which is more than any other oil. Olive oil, as well as light olive oil, is the oil I use in the recipes in this book. Light olive oil is not lower calorie—it has the same amount of calories per tablespoon, 14, as regular olive oil—but rather it has a milder flavor. I use it in baking recipes where the richness of fat contributes to the overall taste, but without the distinctive flavor. Although I generally just call for olive oil, you can use the more flavorful extra-virgin oil in the salads.

Omega-3 essential fatty acids. These polyunsaturated fatty acids are called "essential" because they are important to many body functions, and their anti-inflammatory benefits are crucial to overall body health. Since these acids are not produced by the body, they must be derived from food sources. The best and richest sources are fish, especially those with dark-colored, oily flesh, such as salmon, mackerel, tuna, sardines, and herring (for discussion of PCBs and mercury in fish, see page 189). Dark green leafy vegetables and avocados are nonanimal sources of omega-3s, but they have much less concentrated levels. While there is evidence that omega-3s do have an effect in the prevention and treatment of heart disease, there is no clear-cut evidence that such a relationship exists between omega-3s and prostate cancer. However, a handful of studies suggest that regular consumption of fish may reduce the risk of prostate cancer.

Organic sugar. When sugar cane juice extracted from organically grown sugar cane is dehydrated, the result is a sugar that retains its natural vitamins and minerals. The sugar, with its hint of molasses flavor, can be substituted for the more refined white sugar. Some brand names are Sucanat and Florida Crystals.

Phytochemicals. These plant substances are thought to have disease-fighting capabilities. Phytonutrients, also phyochemicals, have the added advantage of possessing some nutritional value. Phytochemicals may act as antioxidants, alter estrogen metabolism, cause cancer cells to die (apoptosis), and repair DNA damage. Fruits, vegetables, grains, legumes, nuts, soy, and teas are rich sources of phytochemicals.

Phytoestrogens. These phytochemicals are found in plants and behave in some ways like estrogen in the body. As a result, they may help protect against hormone-sensitive cancers, such as prostate and breast. Isoflavones, which include daidzein and genistein, are phytoestrogens and are found in soy products, and ligans, another phytoestrogen, are found in soybeans and whole grains.

Pomegranate juice. The pomegranate is a powerhouse of antioxidants. For centuries in the Middle East and India, the fruit itself has been used to treat different types of inflammation, including sore throats. Some doctors now suggest that a daily glass of pomegranate juice may retard the growth of prostate cancer after the primary treatment of either surgery or radiation. The study, conducted at UCLA, was based on a very small sampling of men, so the results are far from conclusive. Pomegranate juice can be found in the produce section of many supermarkets, and pomegranate juice concentrate is available in health food stores and in the international food section of some supermarkets.

Selenium. This trace mineral performs several functions in the body: It acts as an antioxidant, boosts the immune system, helps fight off infection, and is thought to have prostate cancer–fighting properties. The RDA for selenium is 70 mcg for men, an amount that is usually obtained from a normal, balanced diet. Brazil nuts are selenium rich—a single nut contains about 120 mcg. Other sources include seafood, oats, brown rice, barley, and mushrooms. The concentration of selenium in all these sources depends on the amount of selenium in the soil where the plants are grown, and in some parts of the country, especially the Southeast, the soil is known to be deficient. For a possible positive impact on prostate cancer, some doctors suggest a daily supplement of 200 mcg. There is a danger of toxicity from overdosing on the supplement, so some doctors advise men to take a blood test to measure selenium levels before starting the supplement.

Soy. Soybeans offer a complete protein, which contains all the amino acids essential to human nutrition, without the saturated fat and cholesterol that accompanies animal-based protein. In addition, soybeans are a good source of calcium, iron, zinc, phosphorus, magnesium, B vitamins, omega-3 fatty acids, and soluble fiber. There is some evidence, but certainly not conclusive, that once a man is diagnosed with prostate cancer, soy may lower his risk of developing advanced prostate cancer and lower the risk of dying from the disease. The FDA recommends 25 grams of soy protein a day as part of a heart-healthy diet low in saturated fat and cholesterol.

Soy Protein Content

FOOD	SERVING SIZE	SOY PROTEIN (GRAMS)
Tofu, baked	2 ounces	12
Soybeans, fresh green	$\frac{1}{2}$ cup	11.1
Soy milk, nonfat	1 cup	6.7
Soy yogurt	1 cup	5–8
Tofu, firm	2 ounces	4.7
Tofu, silken	2 ounces	2.7
Soy cheese	1 ounce	2–7

As you increase the amount of soy in your diet, you may experience some stomach and intestinal gas. To avoid this, a smart strategy is to gradually increase the number of soy products you eat over a period of a couple of weeks until you reach the level you're aiming for.

Soy Products. When shopping for soy products, always read the labels. When available, purchase products made with soybeans that are organically grown and not genetically modified.

Soy Cheese

The varieties of soy cheese are increasing, and the quality is improving. Incorporating these cheeses into your cooking allows you to create cholesterol-free and, in some cases, dairy-free and reduced-fat variations of your favorite dishes, such as macaroni and cheese (page 180), pizzas (pages 226–229), and cheese enchiladas (page 171). Since most soy cheeses contain casein, a milk protein that makes for better melting properties, they don't qualify for a dairy-free diet. There are vegan soy cheeses that are dairy-free, but they are not great "melters."

The varieties of cheese available include cheddar, Monterey Jack, jalapeño Jack, feta, queso blanco, grated Parmesan, a variety of smoked cheeses, and mozzarella. In most cases the mozzarella still needs some work, although Follow Your Heart brand has developed a good vegan version. For the others, the brand that I like is Yves Veggie Cuisine. I especially like their grated Parmesan, which I sprinkle on everything from salads and pasta sauces to blanched vegetables and sandwich fillers.

Soy Cream Cheese

I use this occasionally when I want the creaminess of cream cheese in a dessert like cheesecake (page 298) or tiramisu (page 303). It is dairy-free but high-calorie because of the fat, which is not saturated but a combination of monounsaturated and polyunsaturated. It also contains partially hydrogenated vegetable oil, which is a trans fat, so I use it very sparingly. The brand I like is Tofutti.

Soy Yogurt

Use this in place of regular dairy yogurt, in spreads, soups, salad dressings, and baking and for other desserts. The color is slightly gray, and that really is the only drawback. I like Nancy's Cultured Soy when I can find it; otherwise I buy WholeSoy Creamy Cultured Soy because I like its loose consistency. Individual serving sizes of cultured soy are available in a variety of flavors for snacking.

Soy Milk

Soy milk can be substituted for whole milk in most recipes. Producers in this country over the years have managed to eliminate the soybean flavor that is more characteristic of Asian soy milks. The benefit of soy milk is that it is cholesterol-free and dairy-free and provides soy protein and isoflavones. Full-fat soy milk has about the same amount of fat as cow's milk, but the fat is mostly polyunsaturated and monounsaturated. Soy milk is usually calcium and vitamin fortified, providing about 30 percent of the daily requirement for calcium and vitamin D, which can be important for a man if he is at risk for osteoporosis. Soy milk labeled regular or original rather than unsweetened will contain more sugar and, as a result, more calories. Always read the label on the container since calories, fat, and protein will vary according to type and brand.

Canned Soybeans

Yellow and black soybeans are available canned. Use them directly from the can, including the gelled bean juice, for chili, soups, beans and franks (page 170), and salads.

Meat Alternatives

There is a wide range of soy-based meat alternatives available, and some are used in recipes in this book, especially in the sandwich chapter. Read the labels carefully to check the amount of soy protein, fat, and sodium. Soy crumbles resemble ground meat and come packaged in a variety of flavors, such as Tex-Mex and Italian. They can be used as a meat replacement in sloppy Joes (page 77), meatloaf, chili, and tacos. Also available are soy-based meatballs (I make my own—page 178), chickenlike cutlets (page 80), and sausages that include patties and links, chorizo (page 107), hot Italian, and pepperoni. You'll also find soy bacon in a variety of forms, including strips and Canadian bacon rounds.

And then, of course, there is the whole range of veggie burgers, hot dogs, and luncheon meats that run the gamut from bologna and turkey slices to Philly cheese steak slices and pastrami. Sample the different brands to see which you like.

Tofu. Add mineral salts to soy milk to coagulate it, then heat the mixture, and eventually you will produce bean curd or tofu, much in the same way that cheese is made from curds and whey. Tofu comes in water-filled tubs in the refrigerator section in the supermarket, and depending how much water has been pressed from the curd itself during processing, it will be labeled silken, soft, firm, or extra-firm. The tubs will be 14, 16, or sometimes even 19 ounces, depending on the brand and firmness. Tofu can also be found in aseptic boxes, usually 12.3 ounces, and these are generally labeled silken, with an additional labeling of soft, firm, or extra-firm. The silken in the boxes is always smooth and custardlike, and the soft kind has the same texture as the silken tofu in the tubs. The silken firm tofu in boxes is still custardlike, but it can be sliced or chopped as well as pureed. And the silken extra-firm in the box can be stir-fried.

Following are general guidelines for when to use the different types of tofu.

Soft silken tofu is easily pureed and can be used in dressings, soups, sauces, smoothies, cheesecakes, tiramisu, or other desserts where you want a creamy texture.

Soft tofu works well in spreads, and it can replace eggs in a quiche or scrambled eggs (page 271), or cheese in stuffed pasta shells or other pasta dishes.

Firm tofu is ideal for stir-fries, stews where the tofu needs to hold its shape during simmering, and even for kebabs when barbecuing.

Extra-firm tofu has a texture similar to feta cheese. It can be sliced, diced, and stir-fried.

Baked and smoked tofu are first marinated and then cooked. The tofu can be sliced and diced and added to salads and stir-fries.

Although there are "lite" and "fat-free" tofu varieties, the change in texture doesn't justify the very small savings in calories.

Turmeric. Spill a little of this spice on a kitchen counter or on your clothes, and you'll probably have to bleach it out. Ground from the root of a plant in the ginger family, turmeric has been used for thousands of years in Asian cooking and to dye cloth. It imparts a vivid yellow color to any dish. Look at the label on a jar of curry powder and hot dog mustard, and you'll find it listed. Turmeric tastes slightly bitter and astringent. Curcumin, the yellow pigment in turmeric, is thought to have medicinal qualities. In fact, the purported antioxidant, anti-inflammatory, and anticarcinogenic properties of curcumin have been the subject of studies at the M. D. Anderson cancer center in Texas and the Memorial Sloan-Kettering Cancer Center in New York City. But for the moment, turmeric remains in that hazy category of "home remedies."

Vitamin E. This fat-soluble vitamin is thought to act as an antioxidant in the body to prevent cell damage caused by free radicals resulting from a cell's natural metabolism. Recent studies have questioned the effectiveness of vitamin E as a supplement, at least as related to cardiovascular disease, and what the appropriate dosage may be. A long term trial (SELECT), scheduled to be completed at the beginning of the next decade, is measuring whether 400 IU of vitamin E a day can reduce the risk of prostate cancer. For prostate health (before and after diagnosis), some doctors recommend 200 to 400 IU of vitamin E a day, with mixed tocopherols, including d-gamma. Consult your doctor about this.

CHAPTER II

SNACKS & DRINKS

ONE OF THE KEYS TO REALLY HEALTHY EATING (and preventing and battling prostate cancer as well as cardiovascular disease) is getting a handle on snacking—that means keeping it low-calorie and low-fat. Just take a walk through the supermarket aisles and see how much space is devoted to those easy-to-open boxes and bags of salty and sugary munchies, and the role that snacking plays in our culture becomes evident. It is clearly a contributing cause to the problems of overweight and obesity.

Probably the best strategy is to remove temptation. What I've done is to just empty my refrigerator and cupboards of certain items: hunks of cheese, cheese straws, cookies, ice cream, and on and on. And because I'm fairly rigorous about my eating, I try to avoid items that contain dairy, saturated fat, and hydrogenated oils (with the very infrequent exception of soy cream cheese in desserts).

I've also discovered that if I have a parade of sensible snacks throughout the day, I tend to eat much less at regular meals. This eliminates the hazard of binge eating when driven by hunger pangs—that's the danger zone. Healthy snacking keeps my energy level relatively uniform and constant throughout the day. And there are no excessive highs or lows from eating too much food at one sitting. When there's no time to stop for a sensible meal, it's tempting to take the easy way out, filling up on high-fat, high-sugar snacks, all empty calories. And beware of those store-bought snacks claiming no fat—they frequently assault you with a huge amount of empty calories.

For the no-prep snack, fruit is the easy fix, usually providing a range of antioxidants and fiber as well as vitamins and minerals. The choices usually include oranges, apples, bananas, and dried fruit such as apricots and cranberries. Plus, I always try to keep on hand a cut-up fruit salad: watermelon and papaya, two good sources of lycopene, along with strawberries and blueberries when in season.

There is usually a supply of Brazil nuts as well as unsalted dry-roasted soy nuts in my refrigerator for snacking. The Brazil nuts are an excellent source of selenium, as well as B vitamins and vitamin E, and the soy nuts are rich in soy protein and fiber. Since both nuts do contain a high percentage of fat, and consequently calories, they, like most things, should be eaten in moderation. Most of the fat, however, is monounsaturated and polyunsaturated, which have been shown to lower blood cholesterol levels.

Since I do most of my work at home, I make sure to always have on hand a couple of homemade items, so when I need a break or start to get a little hungry, it's a quick trip to the kitchen. If a snack also can travel well, then I throw it into the car when I run errands so there is less temptation when on the road to pull into you know where. Some of my favorite travel snacks are: Baked Trail Mix with Dried Cranberries (page 68) with almost 4 grams of fiber per serving, Salsa-Marinated Vegetables with Coriander (page 60), with lots of antioxidants at less than 100 calories per serving, and Spicy Roasted Edamame (page 63), rich in soy protein and fiber.

I like versatility in my snacks, and the Dips and Spreads section capitalizes on that trait. Many of the very low-fat and low-calorie combinations, such as Tuna and White Bean Spread with Lemon and Rosemary (page 46), Black Bean Dip with Cilantro and Lime (page 43), and Sun-Dried Tomato Dip (page 47) are easily scooped up with low-fat Homemade Pita Chips (page 53), or spread on whole-grain bread as a sandwich filler. The Black Olive Spread with Sun-Dried Tomatoes (page 44) adds a tasty zing to salads and is an excellent topper for pasta or baked fish such as cod. All of these can be spread on Spicy Flat Bread (page 54) or low-fat crackers, and they perform very well as appetizers when accompanied with cut-up fresh vegetables. Although there is a wide variety of good-quality dips available in the refrigerator section of the supermarket and I do use them in a pinch, I still like to make my own so I can control the ingredients that I use.

For a more substantial snack, try crostini (page 56), or little toasts, spread with a flavorful topping such as Roasted Red Pepper Dip (page 50), a great source of vitamin C and antioxidants, or caramelized onion (page 57)—and these are practically fat-free, with only about 25 calories per serving. And to underscore the versatility factor, some of these toppings work well as quick pasta sauces.

As an introduction to tofu, an important source of plant protein and isoflavones, thought to have prostate cancer-fighting properties, there are Tofu Snack Triangles with Ginger and Honey (page 64) and Susan's Marinated Five-Spice Tofu (page 65). There is fat in tofu, but it's the heart-healthy polyunsaturated and monounsaturated kinds.

In our diet-cola culture, good-tasting beverages with important health benefits are usually overlooked or not even considered. Three standards in my repertoire are Blueberry-OJ Smoothie (page 69), Watermelon-Banana Smoothie (page 69), and Thai-Style Tomato Cocktail (page 71), a lycopene treasure, delicious cold or warm, with or without vodka.

Get a grip on snacking, and you've made a good beginning toward a prostate-savvy diet.

Black Bean Dip with Cilantro and Lime

You would never guess this rich-tasting, lime-accented dip is practically fat-free. And, the two kinds of beans provide almost 3 grams of protein and 3 grams of fiber per quarter cup.

Serving Suggestions: Spoon the back bean mixture into a small bowl and accompany with cut-up raw vegetables and cumin- or chili-flavored pita chips (page 53) for scooping. Or, for an instant snack, spread it over small, reduced-fat flour tortillas, roll up, and warm in a microwave or 350°F conventional oven.

MAKES ABOUT 3 CUPS
Prep: 15 minutes / Refrigerate: 2 hours

> 1 can (15 ounces) black beans, drained and rinsed
> 1 can (15.5 ounces) chickpeas, drained and rinsed
> $\frac{1}{4}$ cup vegetable broth, homemade (page 101) or store-bought
> 2 cloves garlic, coarsely chopped
> 2 tablespoons coarsely chopped red onion
> $\frac{1}{2}$ small red bell pepper, cored, seeded, and coarsely chopped
> 2 tablespoons freshly squeezed lime juice
> $\frac{1}{3}$ cup coarsely chopped fresh cilantro
> $\frac{1}{4}$ teaspoon salt
> $\frac{1}{8}$ teaspoon black pepper

1. In a food processor, combine black beans, chickpeas, and broth with on-and-off pulses until mixed but not pureed. Add garlic, red onion, and bell pepper, and pulse to mix. Add lime juice, cilantro, salt, and black pepper, and process until chunky.

2. Scrape into a small bowl and refrigerate, covered, for 2 hours to allow flavors to mellow.

Make-Ahead Tip: Dip can be refrigerated for up to three days.

Black Olive Spread with Sun-Dried Tomatoes

Always keep a jar of this mixture on hand because it's great for adding flavor to a whole range of dishes. Even though the olives contribute fat, remember it's the good kind of fat, monounstaurated, and not the saturated variety from animals. And the sun-dried tomatoes provide a healthy amount of the antioxidant lycopene.

Serving Suggestions: Accompany with Spicy Flat Bread (page 54), Homemade Pita Chips (page 53), Homemade Crostini (page 56), or cut-up fresh vegetables such as red bell pepper, fennel, carrots, and broccoli. Use as a sandwich spread with sliced tomatoes and watercress or arugula on slices of whole-grain bread. Spread over a fish fillet, such as blue-fish, cod, or halibut, and then bake. Toss with a whole-wheat pasta such as penne or rotelle and cherry tomatoes to create a flavorful entree. And try stirring a tablespoon or two of the spread into a vegetable soup, or tossing it with cooked vegetables, such as broccoli or green beans.

MAKES ABOUT 1 CUP
Prep: 10 minutes

> 6 large pieces sun-dried tomatoes packed in oil, blotted dry with paper towels
>
> 2 cloves garlic, finely chopped
>
> 1 cup pitted oil-cured black olives (Greek and Italian are both good choices)
>
> 2 tablespoons capers, drained (optional)
>
> 2 tablespoons olive oil
>
> 1 tablespoon freshly squeezed lemon juice, or to taste

1. In a small food processor or blender, pulse together sun-dried tomatoes and garlic until evenly combined and coarsely chopped. Add olives, capers if using, and oil and pulse until spread is evenly mixed but still has a coarse texture.

2. Add lemon juice, a little at a time, until the flavor of the spread is as perky as you want.

Make-Ahead Tip: Spread can be refrigerated for up to five days.

Edamame and Chickpea Dip with Lemon

This dip takes its inspiration from hummus, the classic Middle Eastern chickpea spread, and mixes in edamame for their beneficial isoflavones, which are believed to have prostate cancer–fighting properties. The flavor can be endlessly varied by adding ground cumin, chili powder, dried basil, dried rosemary, dried thyme, or fresh mint, fresh basil, or fresh thyme. For a crowd, this recipe is easily doubled.

Serving Suggestions: For dipping, accompany with Homemade Pita Chips (page 53) or a variety of cut-up vegetables such as carrots, broccoli, and green beans. Spread it on whole-grain crispy flat bread for a snack or on slices of whole-grain bread and top with lettuce and tomato for a delicious sandwich.

MAKES $1\frac{2}{3}$ CUPS
Prep: 10 minutes / Refrigerate: 2 hours

  1 cup frozen shelled and blanched edamame
  1 cup canned chickpeas, rinsed and drained
  1 small scallion, trimmed and cut into 1-inch pieces, plus additional, thinly sliced,
    for garnish
  2 tablespoons olive oil or tahini (sesame paste)
  2 tablespoons freshly squeezed lemon juice
  2 tablespoons edamame cooking liquid or water
  $\frac{1}{2}$ teaspoon salt
  Large pinch cayenne, or more to taste
  Sprinkle of paprika, for garnish

1. Cook edamame according to package directions. Drain well and set aside to cool.
2. In a food processor, combine edamame, chickpeas, scallion, olive oil, lemon juice, water, salt, and cayenne. Process until smooth, 1 to 2 minutes, scraping down sides of bowl as needed.
3. Spoon into serving dish and garnish with sprinkling of paprika.

Make-Ahead Tip: Dip can be refrigerated for up to three days.

Variation: Edamame and Chickpea Dip with Lemon and Roasted Red Pepper: Add 1 cup drained, bottled roasted red pepper to processor in step 2. Makes $2\frac{1}{4}$ cups.

White Bean Spread with Balsamic Vinegar and Rosemary

This practically fat-free spread, with almost 1 gram of fiber per tablespoon, is amazingly versatile—take a look at the variations that follow. For the rosemary you can substitute other dried herbs and spices such as basil, tarragon, curry powder, ground cumin, or ground fennel. If you're a garlic lover, include the optional clove.

Serving Suggestions: For snacking or an appetizer, serve with raw vegetables or Homemade Pita Chips (page 53) for dipping. Or spread over small pieces of plain or toasted multigrain bread or Homemade Crostini (page 56) and top with very thin slices of plum tomato or bottled roasted red bell peppers and a sprinkle of chopped parsley or cilantro. For an instant soup, stir in vegetable broth until it's the desired consistency.

MAKES ABOUT 1 CUP

Prep: 10 minutes

$\frac{1}{4}$ cup coarsely chopped red onion, or 3 scallions, trimmed and sliced

1 clove garlic, halved (optional)

1 can (15 ounces) cannellini beans, drained and rinsed

2 teaspoons balsamic vinegar, or freshly squeezed lemon juice

1 teaspoon olive oil

$\frac{1}{2}$ teaspoon dried rosemary, crumbled

$\frac{1}{4}$ teaspoon salt

$\frac{1}{8}$ teaspoon black pepper

1. In a food processor, finely chop onion and garlic, if using.

2. Add beans, vinegar, oil, rosemary, salt, and pepper. Puree until smooth and well combined.

3. Scrape into a refrigerator container and, for best flavor, refrigerate for 2 hours.

Make-Ahead Tip: Spread can be refrigerated for up to three days.

Variations: Herbed White Bean Spread with Balsamic Vinegar: In step 1, add $\frac{1}{4}$ cup fresh flat-leaf parsley leaves and $\frac{1}{4}$ cup fresh basil leaves. Makes about 1 cup.

Tuna and White Bean Spread with Lemon and Rosemary: In step 1, add a 6-ounce can solid white tuna packed in water, drained, and $\frac{1}{2}$ cup fresh flat-leaf parsley leaves. Use 1 tablespoon freshly squeezed lemon juice instead of vinegar. Makes about $1\frac{1}{2}$ cups.

White Bean Spread with Tahini and Rosemary: In step 2, add 2 tablespoons tahini (sesame paste) and 1 tablespoon freshly squeezed lemon juice instead of vinegar. Makes about 1 cup.

Sun-Dried Tomato Dip

There are only four ingredients in this dip, which is rich in the antioxidant lycopene.

Serving Suggestions: Raw vegetables are good for dippers. Spread on whole-grain crackers, use as a sandwich spread, or swirl a little into Tomato and Red Bell Pepper Soup with Basil (page 100).

MAKES ABOUT $1\frac{1}{2}$ CUPS
Prep: 5 minutes

1 can (15 ounces) cannellini beans, drained and rinsed
1 tablespoon olive oil
8 large pieces sun-dried tomato, packed in oil, blotted dry with paper towels
$\frac{1}{4}$ cup vegetable broth, homemade (page 101) or store-bought, plus additional if desired

In a food processor, combine beans, oil, and tomato pieces. Process until mixture is coarsely combined. Add broth and process to a smooth paste. For a thinner dip, add more broth until desired consistency.

Make-Ahead Tip: Dip can be refrigerated for up to three days.

Herbed Cheese Spread with Sun-Dried Tomatoes

When I want the taste of cream cheese in a recipe, I turn to an imitation version. There are two soy substitutes for cream cheese that I like: one is Tofutti brand, and the other is SoyBoy. But try all the brands, and then you can decide for yourself. Also be aware that there is a small amount of partially hydrogenated soybean oil in the cream cheese, and that the product is high in fat with some saturated fat. Soy-based mayonnaise is an excellent product and works well in all the places where you would use regular mayo. You can easily double or triple this recipe for a larger crowd.

Serving Suggestions: For an appetizer or snack, try spread on all kinds of crackers or cut-up vegetables. Use to make Ham and Herbed Cheese Roll-Up sandwiches (page 84) or other sandwiches, such as sliced tomato with lettuce. You can substitute dried dill for the basil, if you like.

MAKES $\frac{1}{2}$ CUP
Prep: 5 minutes

  4 ounces chive-flavored soy cream cheese

  2 tablespoons finely chopped oil-packed sun-dried tomatoes

  1 tablespoon eggless soy-based mayonnaise

  $\frac{1}{2}$ teaspoon dried basil

  $\frac{1}{4}$ teaspoon Dijon mustard

  $\frac{1}{8}$ teaspoon salt

  $\frac{1}{8}$ teaspoon black pepper

In a small bowl, stir together all the ingredients until well blended.

Make-Ahead Tip: Spread can be refrigerated for up to five days.

Green Goddess Dip with Edamame

Here a favorite American salad dressing is transformed into a dip. Edamame and soy yogurt are sources of isoflavones, thought to have prostate cancer–fighting properties. To transform the dip back into a dressing, thin it with a little unsweetened soy milk or water to the desired consistency. Taste and adjust seasoning, adding additional lemon juice, if needed. If fresh mint or tarragon is not available, substitute the dried version to taste, starting with about a half teaspoon. But the fresh does make for a more vibrant flavor.

Serving Suggestions: Arrange a platter of cherry tomatoes, small broccoli and cauliflower florets, radishes, carrot sticks, and blanched green beans for dipping.

MAKES $1\frac{1}{2}$ CUPS
Prep: 10 minutes / Cook: 5 minutes

> 1 cup frozen shelled and blanched edamame
> $\frac{1}{4}$ cup fresh parsley leaves
> 2 tablespoons coarsely chopped fresh mint leaves
> 2 tablespoons fresh tarragon leaves
> 1 scallion (green part only), trimmed and cut into $\frac{1}{2}$-inch pieces
> $\frac{1}{2}$ cup plain soy yogurt
> 2 tablespoons freshly squeezed lemon juice
> $1\frac{1}{2}$ teaspoons anchovy paste (optional)
> $\frac{1}{4}$ teaspoon salt
> $\frac{1}{8}$ teaspoon black pepper
> $\frac{1}{2}$ cup eggless soy-based mayonnaise

1. Cook edamame according to package directions. Drain well.

2. In a small food processor or blender, combine parsley, mint, tarragon, and scallion. Process until finely chopped. Transfer to a small bowl and set aside.

3. Add edamame and yogurt to the processor. Process until well blended, 1 to 2 minutes. Add lemon juice, anchovy paste if using, salt, pepper, mayonnaise, and reserved chopped herbs. Process just until mixture is combined. Scrape into a bowl and serve.

Make-Ahead Tip: Dip can be refrigerated for up to two days.

Roasted Red Pepper Dip

You'll get a healthy dose of antioxidants with this practically fat-free dip. The curry variation that follows includes silken tofu for a creamier texture.

Serving Suggestions: Serve with Homemade Pita Chips (page 53), spoon onto crackers, spread in sandwiches instead of mayonnaise, use as a dip with raw vegetables, or swirl a tablespoon or two into a vegetable or bean soup. This is also delicious tossed with cooked vegetables such as green beans or summer squash.

MAKES 1 CUP
Prep: 10 minutes

1 jar (12 ounces) roasted red peppers, drained and blotted dry with paper towels

2 teaspoons olive oil

1 tablespoon balsamic vinegar or freshly squeezed lemon juice

$\frac{1}{4}$ teaspoon salt

$\frac{1}{8}$ teaspoon black pepper

1. In a food processor, with on-and-off pulses, finely chop red pepper.

2. Add oil, vinegar, salt, and pepper and process just until almost incorporated—the trick is to not overprocess the mixture.

Make-Ahead Tip: Dip can be refrigerated for up to three days.

Variation: Roasted Red Pepper and Chutney Spread with Curry: In a small, dry, nonstick skillet, toast 2 teaspoons curry powder over medium-low heat, stirring occasionally, until fragrant, about 2 minutes. In step 1, add curry powder; 4 scallions, trimmed and sliced; 1 tablespoon sherry vinegar or red wine vinegar instead of balsamic; $\frac{1}{4}$ cup mango chutney, any large pieces chopped; and 4 ounces silken tofu. Proceed with rest of recipe. Makes about $1\frac{3}{4}$ cups.

Thai-Style Dipping Sauce with Cilantro

Hidden in this dipping sauce is a little lycopene from the tomato paste. If you happen to have Thai or Vietnamese fish sauce in your cupboard, substitute about a teaspoon of that for the anchovy.

Serving Suggestions: Use as a dipping sauce for cut-up fresh vegetables for snacking, sparingly as a salad dressing, or as an accompaniment with Steamed Fish in Lettuce Wraps (page 211). Or toss a little with cooked vegetables as a side dish.

MAKES ABOUT 1 CUP
Prep: 15 minutes

1 tablespoon tomato paste

1 canned anchovy fillet

1 clove garlic, finely chopped

Juice of 2 limes (generous $\frac{1}{4}$ cup)

2 tablespoons rice wine vinegar, or white wine vinegar

2 tablespoons grated onion

1 tablespoon sugar

1 tablespoon soy sauce

$\frac{1}{8}$ to $\frac{1}{4}$ teaspoon crushed red pepper flakes

2 tablespoons finely chopped fresh cilantro

1. In a small bowl, using the back of a spoon, mash together tomato paste, anchovy, and garlic. Stir in $\frac{1}{2}$ cup water, lime juice, vinegar, onion, sugar, soy sauce, and pepper flakes.
2. Pour the mixture into a small saucepan and heat just to boiling. Remove from heat and stir in cilantro. Let cool to room temperature.

Make-Ahead Tip: Sauce can be refrigerated for up to two days.

Mexican Tomato Salsa with Serrano Chile

This fresh salsa, rich in antioxidants, is from a cookbook that I co-authored, *Modern Mexican Flavors* (Stewart, Tabori & Chang, 2002), by Richard Sandoval, a chef-owner of several restaurants around the country. Richard likes to use honey to sweetly balance the spicy chiles in his cooking.

Serving Suggestions: Accompany with Homemade Tortilla Chips (page 55) or good-quality store-bought low-fat chips. You can also spoon the salsa over broiled fish or steamed vegetables for extra zip.

MAKES ABOUT 2 CUPS
Prep: 10 minutes / Stand: 30 minutes

> 2 tomatoes, cored, seeded, and diced
> $\frac{1}{4}$ cup chopped white onion
> 1 to 2 fresh serrano chiles, stemmed, seeded, and chopped
> 1 tablespoon chopped fresh cilantro
> 2 teaspoons freshly squeezed lemon juice
> 2 teaspoons honey
> $\frac{1}{2}$ teaspoon salt
> $\frac{1}{4}$ teaspoon black pepper

In a medium-size bowl, combine all the ingredients. Let sit for 30 minutes before serving.

Make-Ahead Tip: Salsa can be refrigerated for up to three days.

Homemade Pita Chips

Make a batch of these almost fat-free chips and keep them handy for easy snacking. They're a delicious alternative to commercial crackers, which often are full of hydrogenated fat. And don't be fooled by the commercial reduced-fat or nonfat versions—they usually have added sugar and salt to boost the flavor. See the herb and spice variations that follow.

Serving Suggestions: Use as a scoop for any of the spreads or dips in this chapter for satisfying snacking. Crumble them over grain- or bean-based soups to add crunch.

MAKES 32 CHIPS
Prep: 10 minutes / Cook: 12 minutes

> Nonstick olive oil cooking spray
>
> 2 thin regular-size whole-wheat or other whole-grain pita breads
>
> 1 clove garlic, cut in half lengthwise (optional)

1. Place racks in upper and lower thirds of oven. Heat oven to 375°F. Coat two large baking sheets with nonstick cooking spray.

2. Split each pita bread into two rounds. Rub the rough side of each disk with the cut side of garlic clove, if using. Cut each disk into eight wedges. Place in a single layer on baking sheets.

3. Bake until lightly browned and crisp, 10 to 12 minutes total, switching positions of sheets halfway through baking. Transfer chips to a wire rack and let cool.

Make-Ahead Tip: Chips can be stored, tightly covered, at room temperature, for up to a week.

Herb and Spice Variations: Before baking, sprinkle the chips with dried rosemary, dried thyme, dried tarragon, dried oregano, ground cumin, chili powder, curry powder, ground coriander, or any other favorite herb or spice.

Spicy Flat Bread

The whole-grain flour in this nearly fat-free flat bread adds extra nutrients as well as a slightly sweet, nutty flavor. For a milder taste, omit the red pepper flakes. In the early 1990s, while I was a contributing editor at *Family Circle* magazine, I edited *The Family Circle Cookbook: New Tastes for New Times* (Simon & Schuster, 1992). This recipe is borrowed from that book.

Serving Suggestions: Practically any spread works on these crackers. And if you're looking for something crunchy to go with a salad or a soup, this is your bet.

MAKES ABOUT 40 PIECES
Prep: 20 minutes / Rise: 40 minutes / Cook: 12–15 minutes

$2/3$ cup warm water (105–115°F)

$1/2$ teaspoon sugar

1 teaspoon active dry yeast

$1\frac{1}{4}$ cups all-purpose flour

$1/2$ cup rye or whole-wheat flour

$1/2$ teaspoon salt

Nonstick olive oil cooking spray

1 tablespoon olive oil

1 clove garlic, finely chopped

$1/4$ teaspoon crushed red pepper flakes

1 small red onion, thinly sliced (optional)

1. In a glass measuring cup, stir together water and sugar. Sprinkle yeast over top and let stand until foamy, about 5 minutes. Stir to dissolve yeast.

2. In a food processor, pulse together all-purpose flour, rye flour, and salt until blended. With machine running, pour yeast mixture through top of processor, and then continue to process for 30 seconds to knead dough.

3. Lightly coat a medium-size bowl with cooking spray. Scrape dough into bowl and turn to coat. Cover with a clean kitchen cloth and let rise in a warm place until doubled in volume, about 40 minutes.

4. When almost ready to bake, heat oven to 375°F. Lightly coat two baking sheets with nonstick cooking spray.

5. Divide dough in half. On a floured work surface, roll out each half into a rectangle about 13 x 10 inches.

6. In a small bowl, stir together oil, garlic, and pepper flakes. Spread over flat bread. If using onion, sprinkle over the tops.

7. Bake until golden, 12 to 15 minutes. Slide breads onto a cutting board. While still hot, cut each into about 20 pieces. Serve hot, warm, or at room temperature.

Make-Ahead Tip: Baked flat bread, without the onion, can be stored in airtight container at room temperature for up to a week. Recrisp in a 250°F oven for 10 to 15 minutes.

Homemade Tortilla Chips

These are easy to make and contain none of the added preservatives and fats usually found in the commercially prepared versions. Use low-fat corn tortillas if available.

Serving Suggestions: These go well with the usual salsa and other dips. For a little added crunch, crumble them over grain- or bean-based soups.

MAKES 24 LARGE CHIPS
Prep: 5 minutes / Cook: 12 minutes

Nonstick olive oil cooking spray
Six 6-inch corn tortillas

1. Heat oven to 400°F. Lightly coat a large baking sheet with cooking spray.
2. Lightly coat each tortilla with cooking spray. Stack tortillas and cut into quarters. Separate the triangles and place on baking sheet.
3. Bake until crisp, about 12 minutes. Remove to a wire rack and let cool.

Make-Ahead Tip: Chips can be stored in an airtight container at room temperature for up to a week.

Spice and Herb Variations: Before baking, sprinkle chips with curry powder, chili powder, ground cumin, dried basil, or cayenne.

Homemade Crostini

Use any kind of "brown" bread for these, such as whole-wheat, twelve-grain, or seven-grain. A small baguette is the perfect size and shape, or if you're using square bread slices, cut the slices diagonally from corner to corner to make four triangles. For the more traditional crostini, the bread is first brushed with a little olive oil.

Serving Suggestions: Use as crunchy base for any of the spreads included in this chapter or for constructing mini sandwiches using sliced tomato, salmon salad (page 81), or tuna fish salad (page 82).

MAKES 16 CROSTINI
Prep: 5 minutes / Cook: 1–2 minutes

> 16 slices bread (about 3 inches wide and $\frac{1}{4}$ inch thick)
> 1 clove garlic, crushed (optional)

1. Heat oven to 350°F.
2. Arrange bread slices in a single layer on a baking sheet.
3. Bake until crisp and lightly browned, 1 to 2 minutes. If you want, rub the browned side with garlic.

Make-Ahead Tip: Toasts can be stored in an airtight container at room temperature for up to a week. Recrisp them in 350°F oven for 1 to 2 minutes.

Crostini with Caramelized Onion and Red Wine

The onion mixture takes a while to cook, but it's the slow cooking that creates the intense flavor and marmalade consistency. Onion is a source of vitamin C and phytochemicals that are believed to fight cancer, and in this recipe, the onions are cooked with a little red wine. Some nutritionists and doctors recommend a glass of red wine a day, since it is thought that the red pigment in grape skins may help battle prostate cancer.

Serving Suggestions: These are a nice accompaniment to tomato soup (page 100). Make a double batch of the onion mixture to have on hand for flavoring soups, stews, or broiled fish. Use the onion topping as a sandwich spread; it's great with a veggie burger or even on a tuna salad sandwich. For a pasta dish, toss a couple of large spoonfuls of it onto whole-wheat rigatoni, along with a tablespoon or two of the pasta water.

MAKES 16 CROSTINI
Prep: 10 minutes / Cook: about 1 hour

> 2 teaspoons olive oil
>
> $1\frac{1}{2}$ pounds sweet or yellow onions, chopped
>
> $\frac{1}{8}$ teaspoon salt
>
> Pinch black pepper
>
> 2 tablespoons organic sugar (evaporated cane juice)
>
> $\frac{1}{4}$ cup dry red wine
>
> 1 tablespoon balsamic vinegar
>
> 1 tablespoon chopped fresh parsley
>
> 1 recipe Homemade Crostini (page 56), or 2 English muffins, split, toasted, and cut into quarters

1. In a large nonstick skillet, heat oil over medium heat. Stir in onions, salt, and pepper. Reduce heat to low. Cover skillet and cook, stirring occasionally, for 20 minutes—onions should be very soft.

2. Sprinkle onions with sugar and stir to combine. Cook, uncovered, stirring occasionally, for 10 minutes. Stir in wine and vinegar and cook, uncovered, stirring occasionally, until mixture is thick and soft, about 30 minutes—watch carefully so onions don't scorch. Remove skillet from heat. Stir in parsley.

3. Spoon about 1 tablespoon over each crostini. Serve warm or at room temperature.

Make-Ahead Tip: Onion topping, without parsley, can be refrigerated for up to three days. Gently rewarm in a nonstick skillet, and then stir in parsley.

Crostini with Roasted Bell Pepper

Broiling the bell peppers yourself makes for a richer flavor. Plus, you can save this recipe for that time of the year when there is an abundance of locally grown peppers and their price drops. For a shortcut, substitute bottled roasted red peppers (see Variations, below). Red bell pepper is a good source of a variety of antioxidants.

Serving Suggestions: These work well as an appetizer and as a crunchy accompaniment to soups. For a pasta dish, toss the red pepper mixture with cooked whole-wheat rotelle, penne, or rigatoni, along with a couple of tablespoons of the pasta cooking water.

MAKES 16 CROSTINI
Prep: 15 minutes / Cook: about 20 minutes

> 2 red or orange or yellow bell peppers, or a combination (see Variations, below)
> 1 teaspoon olive oil
> 1 small onion, finely chopped
> 2 cloves garlic, finely chopped
> $\frac{1}{4}$ teaspoon salt
> $\frac{1}{8}$ teaspoon black pepper
> 1 tablespoon grated Parmesan-style soy cheese
> 1 tablespoon finely chopped fresh parsley or fresh basil
> 1 recipe Homemade Crostini (page 56) or 2 English muffins, split, toasted, and cut
>   into quarters

1. Heat broiler. Broil the whole peppers about 4 inches from heat, turning frequently, until blackened on all sides, about 20 minutes. Transfer peppers to a paper bag and seal. Set aside until peppers cool and skins loosen. Leave broiler on.

2. Meanwhile, in a small nonstick skillet, heat oil over medium heat. Add onion and cook, stirring frequently, until slightly softened, about 3 minutes. And garlic, salt, and pepper and cook, stirring, 1 minute. Remove skillet from heat.

3. With fingers, peel off blackened skin from peppers. Blot peppers dry with paper towels. Halve them lengthwise; remove the stem, core, and seeds; and finely chop. In a small bowl, combine peppers and onion mixture.

4. Spread about 1 tablespoon of pepper mixture over each toast. In a small bowl, combine cheese and parsley. Sprinkle scant $\frac{1}{2}$ teaspoon over each toast. Arrange crostini in single layer on a baking sheet.

5. Broil crostini 4 inches from heat until cheese is melted, 30 to 60 seconds. Serve warm.

Make-Ahead Tip: Red pepper topping can be refrigerated for up to three days.

Variations: Using Bottled Roasted Red Peppers: Substitute 1 jar (12 ounces) roasted red peppers for fresh bell peppers. Drain peppers well and blot dry with paper towels. Finely chop and add to onion mixture in step 3.

Black Olives: Chop $\frac{1}{4}$ cup drained, canned, pitted black olives, or pitted oil-cured olives, and add to bell pepper mixture in step 3.

Salsa-Marinated Vegetables with Coriander

In addition to being a snack rich in antioxidants, these bite-size vegetables make the perfect road food for the car, train, or airplane. Three grams of fiber per serving is the added bonus. Vary the kinds of vegetables to suit your own taste, and depending on what looks the freshest in the market. And adjust the cooking times according to the density of the vegetable.

Serving Suggestions: Snack on the vegetables as is, serve them as a side salad with grain or bean dishes, or toss them into a mixed salad.

MAKES 8 SERVINGS

Prep: 15 minutes / Cook: about 10 minutes / Refrigerate: 3 hours

Marinade:

2 cups vegetable broth, homemade (page 101) or store-bought

$\frac{1}{4}$ cup cider vinegar

$\frac{1}{4}$ cup bottled salsa

3 tablespoons olive oil

2 tablespoons balsamic vinegar

1 tablespoon honey

1 tablespoon dried basil

2 teaspoons ground coriander

1 teaspoon salt

$\frac{1}{2}$ teaspoon black pepper

3 cloves garlic, finely chopped

2 bay leaves

Vegetables:

8 ounces baby carrots

$\frac{1}{2}$ pound small white button mushrooms, stems trimmed and caps cleaned

$\frac{1}{2}$ head cauliflower, trimmed and cut into small florets

1 zucchini, trimmed, halved lengthwise if thick, and cut crosswise into $\frac{1}{4}$-inch-thick slices

1. In a medium-size nonaluminum saucepan, combine marinade ingredients. Bring to a gentle boil.

2. Gently drop carrots into gently boiling marinade and cook just until crunchy-tender, about 3 minutes. Remove with a large slotted spoon or skimmer and place in a large bowl. Drop mushrooms into marinade and cook 1 minute, just to infuse with flavor. Remove to bowl with carrots. Repeat with cauliflower and with zucchini, cooking for about 2 minutes each. Pour marinade over vegetables in the bowl.

3. Refrigerate, covered, for at least 3 hours. To serve, remove vegetables from marinade and discard bay leaves.

Make-Ahead Tip: Vegetables can be refrigerated in marinade for up to three days.

Quesadillas with Tomatoes and Chiles

Tomatoes are a source of lycopene and the soy cheese, isoflavones. There are even phytonutrients in the chiles. There is a wide variety of flavored flour tortillas available, so experiment.

Serving Suggestions: Accompany with an escarole and orange salad for a light lunch or supper.

MAKES 12 WEDGES
Prep: 15 minutes / Cook: 12 minutes

> 1 large tomato, cored, seeded, and finely chopped
>
> $\frac{1}{2}$ teaspoon ground cumin
>
> $\frac{1}{2}$ teaspoon salt
>
> 6 low-fat, chipotle chile and red bell pepper 8-inch flour tortillas, or other flavored tortillas
>
> 1 cup (about 4 ounces) shredded Monterey Jack–style or cheddar cheese–style soy cheese
>
> 1 can (4.5 ounces) chopped mild chiles, drained
>
> 1 tablespoon chopped fresh cilantro
>
> Nonstick olive oil cooking spray

1. Heat oven to 200°F.
2. In a small bowl, stir together tomato, cumin, and salt.
3. Place 3 tortillas on a work surface. Sprinkle each equally with tomato mixture, cheese, chiles, and cilantro. Place remaining tortillas on top and gently press to flatten.
4. Coat a large nonstick skillet with nonstick cooking spray. Heat over medium-high heat. Place one quesadilla at a time in the skillet. Cook until lightly browned on both sides and cheese is melted, about 2 minutes per side. Transfer to baking sheet and place in oven to keep warm. Repeat with remaining quesadillas. To serve, cut each quesadilla into 4 wedges.

Make-Ahead Tip: Quesadilla wedges can be tightly wrapped in plastic wrap and refrigerated for up to two days, or frozen for up to a month. To serve as a snack, reheat in a microwave or 350°F oven.

Spicy Roasted Edamame

Shelled edamame (page 30) are available fresh in the produce section of some supermarkets and health food stores and in the frozen food section. Munch on these for a hit of protein, about 5 grams per quarter cup, as well as isoflavones.

Serving Suggestions: Use for snacking or scatter over soups or salads for a flavorful garnish.

MAKES 1¾ CUPS
Prep: 10 minutes / Cook: 15 minutes

  Nonstick olive oil cooking spray
  1 tablespoon olive oil
  1 tablespoon beaten egg white or liquid egg substitute
  2 teaspoons chili powder
  1 teaspoon ground cumin
  ½ teaspoon dried oregano
  ¼ teaspoon black pepper
  ⅛ teaspoon ground cinnamon (optional)
  2 teaspoons organic sugar (evaporated cane juice)
  1 teaspoon salt
  2 cups shelled fresh edamame or frozen shelled and blanched edamame, thawed and
    blotted dry with paper towels

1. Heat oven to 375°F. Line a baking sheet with aluminum foil and coat the foil with cooking spray. ·

2. In a medium-size bowl, whisk together oil, egg white, chili powder, cumin, oregano, pepper, cinnamon if using, 1 teaspoon of the sugar, and ½ teaspoon of the salt. Add edamame and toss well until evenly coated. Spread in a single layer on the prepared baking sheet.

3. Bake until lightly browned, about 15 minutes, stirring halfway through cooking time. Let cool on the baking sheet on a wire rack.

4. Spoon into a bowl. Just before serving, toss with the remaining 1 teaspoon sugar and ½ teaspoon salt.

Make-Ahead Tip: Edamame can be refrigerated for up to two days.

Tofu Snack Triangles with Ginger and Honey

The honey softens the spicy heat of the fresh ginger in this light snack, which is a great introduction to tofu. One serving provides 8 grams of protein with only 1 gram of saturated fat and 95 calories.

Serving Suggestions: You can wrap the triangles individually in a Napa cabbage leaf and arrange on a platter for an appetizer, or munch as a dressed-up snack. Crumble the tofu over your favorite green leafy salad. For an instant soup, float small cubes in a warm bowl of Basic Vegetable Broth (page 101) or canned vegetable broth.

MAKES 8 SERVINGS

Prep: 10 minutes / Cook: 10 minutes / Marinate: 1–2 hours

1 small clove garlic, finely chopped

2 teaspoons finely chopped, peeled fresh ginger

3 tablespoons regular or reduced-sodium soy sauce

2 tablespoons rice vinegar

2 teaspoons dark sesame oil

1 tablespoon honey

14 ounces firm tofu, drained, blotted dry with paper towels, and halved horizontally

1. In a small bowl, whisk together garlic, ginger, soy sauce, vinegar, $\frac{1}{4}$ cup water, oil, and honey. Pour into a large nonstick skillet just large enough to hold tofu pieces in a single layer. (Do not yet add tofu.) Bring to a boil.

2. Place tofu in a single layer in boiling liquid. Reduce heat to low and simmer 5 minutes. Carefully turn tofu over and simmer 5 minutes longer. Remove pan from heat and let stand for 1 to 2 hours, turning tofu over from time to time.

3. Remove tofu from marinade. Cut each half into quarters, then each quarter into 2 triangles, for total of 16 triangles.

Make-Ahead Tip: Tofu can be refrigerated in a covered container for up to two days.

Susan's Marinated Five-Spice Tofu

This recipe was developed by Susan McQuillan, who has contributed much to this book. It is based on a Korean tofu she often purchases during her shopping trips to New York City's Chinatown. Chinese five-spice powder is a sweet and spicy blend of cinnamon, ginger, cloves, fennel, and star anise. One serving of this snack provides about 6 grams of soy protein.

Serving Suggestions: Dice the tofu and toss with soba noodles and a peanut or sesame sauce, mix with steamed green beans, or add to any Asian-style salad or stir-fry. Or eat as is, with a little chutney on the side for dipping.

MAKES 4 SERVINGS
Prep: 5 minutes / Cook: 10 minutes / Marinate: 1–2 hours

  3 tablespoons regular or reduced-sodium soy sauce
  2 teaspoons molasses
  1 teaspoon Chinese five-spice powder
  1 pound firm tofu, drained and blotted dry with paper towels

1. In a large skillet, combine 1 cup water, soy sauce, molasses, and five-spice powder. Bring to a boil over medium-high heat, stirring to blend.
2. Meanwhile, slice tofu horizontally into $\frac{1}{2}$-inch-thick cakes. Add to the skillet in a single layer. Reduce heat to low and simmer for 5 minutes. Carefully turn tofu cakes over and simmer 5 minutes longer. Remove pan from heat and let stand for 1 to 2 hours, turning tofu cakes over from time to time.
3. Remove tofu from marinade and serve, cutting into smaller pieces as desired.

Make-Ahead Tip: Tofu can be refrigerated in a covered container for up to two days. Refrigerate any remaining marinade and reuse within five days. Dilute with a little water first, before using to season more tofu.

Greek-Style Marinated Tofu

If you're fond of feta, you'll like this marinated tofu as a replacement that is not animal-derived, and thereby avoids cholesterol and saturated fat.

Serving Suggestions: Excellent as a snack with whole-grain flat breads or Homemade Pita Chips (page 53). Toss it into a Greek salad (page 121) or a simple green salad, or gently stir it into hot orzo with pine nuts, or cooked brown rice with chopped scallions and red bell pepper…the possibilities are endless.

MAKES ABOUT 2 CUPS
Prep: 10 minutes / Refrigerate: at least 30 minutes

$\frac{1}{4}$ cup olive oil

2 tablespoons red wine vinegar

1 tablespoon freshly squeezed lemon juice

1 clove garlic, finely chopped

1 teaspoon dried oregano, crumbled

$\frac{1}{4}$ teaspoon salt

$\frac{1}{8}$ teaspoon black pepper

14 ounces firm tofu, drained and blotted dry with paper towels

In a large bowl, whisk together oil, vinegar, lemon juice, garlic, oregano, salt, and pepper. Crumble tofu into bowl and gently stir. Refrigerate for at least 30 minutes.

Make-Ahead Tip: Tofu can be refrigerated in covered container for up to three days.

Pita Pizzas with Roasted Peppers

This recipe provides a reason for exploring the soy-based cheeses available in your health food store or supermarket. The roasted peppers are full of antioxidants, and the tomato sauce is a common source of lycopene. And this protein-rich snack (5 grams) weighs in at only 76 calories with no saturated fat.

Serving Suggestions: To create a meal, serve with a bowl of Cream of Broccoli-Carrot Soup (page 96). For the warmer months, Garden Gazpacho with Edamame (page 112) is a good accompaniment. And a spinach salad makes for an easy side, especially with the availability of prewashed greens in bags.

MAKES 4 SERVINGS

Prep: 10 minutes / Cook: 3 minutes

- $\frac{1}{2}$ cup bottled roasted red bell peppers, blotted dry with paper towels and cut into $\frac{1}{8}$ -inch-wide strips
- $\frac{1}{4}$ teaspoon crushed fennel seeds, or dried oregano, crumbled
- $\frac{1}{4}$ teaspoon salt
- $\frac{1}{8}$ teaspoon black pepper
- 2 small (4-inch) whole-wheat pita breads
- 8 teaspoons bottled meatless marinara sauce, pizza sauce, or Homemade All-Purpose Tomato Sauce (page 259)
- $\frac{1}{2}$ cup (about 2 ounces) shredded mozzarella-style soy cheese
- $\frac{1}{2}$ small red onion, thinly sliced and separated into rings

1. Heat broiler.
2. In a small bowl, combine red pepper, fennel or oregano, salt, and pepper.
3. Separate each pita bread into 2 round halves. Place halves, rough side up, on a baking sheet.
4. Broil pita 4 inches from heat until golden brown around edges, about 1 minute.
5. Spread 2 teaspoons marinara sauce over each pita, covering edges. Spoon 2 tablespoons red pepper mixture over each pita. Sprinkle with cheese, dividing equally among the rounds, then onion.
6. Return pitas to broiler and cook until cheese is melted and pizzas are hot, about 2 minutes.

Baked Trail Mix with Dried Cranberries

Squirrel away small containers of this mix in the kitchen, office, and car, so a snack is just a short reach away. Look for the unsweetened versions of the cereals, and you'll keep the calories down. But keep in mind that, even with unsweetened cereals, a half cup of the mix has 189 calories, although the rest of the nutrition profile is good: 4 grams of fiber, 5 grams of protein, and a large portion of monounsaturated fat, which is thought to be heart-healthy as well as prostate-healthy.

MAKES ABOUT 10 CUPS
Prep: 5 minutes / Cook: 25 minutes

Nonstick olive oil cooking spray

4 cups natural unsweetened multigrain O-shaped cereal

4 cups natural unsweetened multigrain square-shaped cereal

2 cups peanuts or cashew pieces

2 cups dried cranberries

2 tablespoons light olive oil

1 teaspoon curry powder, ground cumin, seasoned salt, or other seasoning (optional)

1. Heat oven to 275°F. Lightly coat two baking pans with nonstick cooking spray.
2. In a large bowl, stir together cereals, nuts, and cranberries. Drizzle oil over top while stirring. Stir in curry powder or other seasoning, if using. Spread evenly in prepared pans.
3. Bake until lightly colored, about 20 to 25 minutes, stirring once after 10 minutes. Let cool in pans on wire racks.

Make-Ahead Tip: Trail mix can be stored in a tightly covered container at room temperature for up to four days.

Watermelon-Banana Smoothie

Watermelon seems to be in the supermarket all year round, and it's an excellent source of lycopene. For a variation, toss a few cubes of fresh papaya into the blender. Papaya is another good source of lycopene.

Serving Suggestions: Great for breakfast, with a sandwich for lunch, or as an afternoon snack.

MAKES 1 SERVING
Prep: 5 minutes

> 1 small ripe banana, peeled and cut into chunks
> $\frac{1}{2}$ cup watermelon cubes, seeds removed (or use seedless melon)
> $\frac{1}{4}$ cup orange juice
> 1 tablespoon freshly squeezed lime juice

In a blender or food processor, puree together all the ingredients. Serve immediately.

Blueberry-OJ Smoothie

Blueberries are considered by some to be a superfood: one serving provides as many antioxidants as five servings of carrots, broccoli, or an orange-fleshed squash. The soy yogurt packs a protein wallop and provides isoflavones. And there are 7 grams of fiber in this drink. You can also substitute strawberries or raspberries for the blueberries.

Serving Suggestions: Works for breakfast, lunch, or snack, and as an accompaniment with a sandwich or bowl of fruit—that last combo will really increase your fruit consumption for the day.

MAKES 1 SERVING
Prep: 5 minutes

> 1 cup plain soy yogurt
> 1 cup blueberries, fresh or frozen
> 1 small ripe banana, peeled
> $\frac{1}{4}$ cup orange juice

In a blender or food processor, puree together all the ingredients. Serve immediately.

Tropical Pink Thick Shake

For an extra-frosty shake, freeze the strawberries and papaya before using. Papaya and strawberries are both good sources of lycopene, and the silken tofu creates a creamy shakelike texture with the added bonus of soy protein and isoflavones.

Serving Suggestions: Breakfast, midafternoon snack, or late night zip—the shake fills any of these needs.

MAKES 2 SERVINGS (ABOUT 2 CUPS)
Prep: 5 minutes

6 ounces silken tofu, blotted dry with paper towels and chilled

8 ripe strawberries, hulled

1 cup papaya or mango chunks

1 cup orange juice, chilled

$\frac{1}{4}$ teaspoon dried mint (optional)

In a blender or food processor, puree together all the ingredients until very smooth. Serve immediately.

Thai-Style Tomato Cocktail

Ginger, lime, sweet onion such as Vidalia, and cilantro spice up this Southeast Asian–style version of the classic Virgin Mary drink. Warm it up on a cold winter's day or serve it over ice in summer. Tomato juice is rich in lycopene.

Serving Suggestions: Sip with a veggie burger or sandwich. If you're mixing for a party, feel free to add a splash of vodka or gin.

MAKES 1 DRINK
Prep: 5 minutes

    6 ounces tomato juice
    1 tablespoon grated sweet onion such as Vidalia
    1 tablespoon freshly squeezed lime juice
    2 teaspoons ginger juice (see Note)
    $\frac{1}{2}$ teaspoon regular or reduced-sodium soy sauce
    Ice cubes (if serving cold)
    Finely chopped fresh cilantro and lime slices, for garnish (optional)

For a cold drink, in an 8-ounce glass combine tomato juice, onion, lime juice, ginger juice, and soy sauce. Add ice and garnish with cilantro and lime slices, if using. For a warm drink, in a small saucepan, combine the first five ingredients and warm gently over low heat. Serve in a mug, garnished with cilantro and lime, if you like.

Note: To make ginger juice, grate a knob or thumb-size piece of unpeeled fresh ginger into a sheet of paper towel. Gather into a bundle and squeeze gently over a small bowl to extract juice. The amount of juice you'll get depends on the freshness of the root—the fresher the root, the more juice. Use leftover ginger juice to flavor lemonade, hot or iced tea, broths, and stir-fry dishes.

CHAPTER III

SANDWICHES

IF SNACKING RATES AS OUR NUMBER-ONE cultural pastime, then sandwich-eating has got to be number two (maybe along with TV watching). And a sandwich fits in well with our multitasking culture: It can be a snack, lunch, dinner, a soup go-with, or the ultimate travel companion.

For the bread, the goal is to use whole-grain products for their added nutrient and fiber benefits. There are the usual whole-wheat and multigrain varieties, but then you can quickly move on to whole-wheat pita, low-fat corn tortillas, low-fat flour tortillas, whole-wheat English muffins, shepherd's bread, spinach or red-pepper sandwich wraps, rice paper, and even Romaine lettuce leaves for sandwich packets.

For instant fillings there is everything from canned vegetarian refried beans and slices of soy cheese to crushed canned cannellini beans. And then for flavor enhancers, the selection is endless: chutneys, flavored ketchups, mustards, bottled pickled ginger, applesauce, eggless soy-based mayonnaise, mustard, adobo sauce from canned chiles in adobo, bottled pesto sauces and olive mixes, and Asian fish sauces, to mention just a few. Take a stroll through the international food aisle and the mustard and relish aisle of your supermarket and check out all the different bottles and jars. But remember, the bottom line is to keep it low in fat, and to work in as many vegetables as possible for their antioxidant properties.

When it comes to the recipes, many diner and deli hits are in this chapter, but in a slightly different garb, using soy-based meat substitutes: Cheese "Steak" Sandwich with Red Bell Pepper (page 75) with only 1 gram of saturated fat, Reuben Sandwich with Sauerkraut and Thousand Island Dressing (page 76) at less than 200 calories and only 1 gram of saturated fat, Sloppy Joes (page 77), and Chili Dog on a Bun (page 78). I've replaced my formerly usual bacon-cheddar burger with a Chickpea Burger with Almonds and Ginger (page 88), and two other nonmeat burgers that incorporate high-fiber beans, antioxidant-intense sweet potatoes, and selenium-rich Brazil nuts. The usual whole-egg-and-mayonnaise-laden tuna salad has been transformed into a lighter tuna salad (page 82) and an omega-3-rich salmon salad (page 81).

"Meatball" Hero with Mozzarella

Here it is—the Italian deli favorite, served open-faced and meant to be eaten with a knife and fork. For an extra kick, sprinkle with crushed red pepper flakes. The meatballs are made with a delicious soy alternative, which introduces isoflavones.

Serving Suggestions: For a salad, toss shredded Romaine lettuce or escarole with a low-fat Italian dressing and top with shredded carrot. Alternatively, the sharp flavor of a vinegar-based coleslaw would complement the rich meatballs.

MAKES 8 PIECES

Prep: 10 minutes / Cook: 2 minutes

  2 cups Homemade All-Purpose Tomato Sauce (page 259), or bottled meatless marinara sauce

  16 Herbed and Parmesan "Meatballs" (page 178)

  2 whole-grain or semolina rolls (about 6 inches long), halved lengthwise and crosswise

  1 cup (4 ounces) shredded mozzarella-style soy cheese

1. In a medium-size saucepan, gently heat together sauce and meatballs until meatballs are heated through.

2. Meanwhile, heat broiler. If rolls are dense, pull out some of the bread from inside to make slight hollows (reserve pulled bread to make bread crumbs or croutons). Place bread, cut-side up, on the broiler pan.

3. Spoon some sauce onto each piece of bread. Top with meatballs, remaining sauce, and cheese.

4. Broil 6 inches from heat until cheese is melted and bread is lightly toasted around edges, 1 to 2 minutes. Serve hot.

Cheese "Steak" Sandwich with Red Bell Pepper

The inspiration for this sandwich is the Philly classic. The bell pepper provides antioxidants and the ketchup brings a smattering of lycopene. Isoflavones come from the soy in the cheese and the "meat" slices. And besides all this, the sandwich is delicious.

But keep in mind that soy alternatives contain quite a bit of sodium—so reserve this sandwich, which contains about 1,200 mg, for the occasional indulgence. However, the sandwich weighs in at only about 250 calories, with 1 gram saturated fat and no cholesterol—and it contains 7 grams of fiber.

Serving Suggestions: How about blanched green beans tossed with sliced, bottled, pickled Italian peppers and a little olive oil for a side salad?

MAKES 4 SANDWICHES
Prep: 10 minutes / Cook: 7 minutes

> 2 teaspoons olive oil
> 1 large sweet onion such as Vidalia, halved and thinly sliced crosswise
> 1 package (6 ounces) Philly cheese steak–style soy slices or pastrami-style soy slices, cut into strips
> 4 whole-grain hot dog–style rolls, split open like a book, or hamburger buns, split
> $\frac{1}{4}$ cup ketchup
> $\frac{1}{2}$ teaspoon dried oregano, crushed
> 8 slices American-style soy cheese
> $\frac{1}{2}$ cup finely chopped red or yellow bell pepper

1. In a large nonstick skillet, heat oil over medium heat. Add onion and cook, stirring occasionally, until softened, about 4 minutes.

2. Add strips of cheese steak–style soy and cook, stirring gently, until heated through, about 1 minute.

3. Meanwhile, lightly toast rolls or buns in a toaster oven or under the broiler. Spread each roll or bottom half of each bun with ketchup and sprinkle with oregano, dividing equally. Top each with 2 cheese slices and return to the toaster to melt. Place rolls on serving plates.

4. Spoon warm onion and soy strips evenly onto buns. Sprinkle with bell pepper. Place tops on bun bottoms, if using buns rather than hot dog rolls. Serve at once.

Reuben Sandwich with Sauerkraut and Thousand Island Dressing

This meatless version is not as decadent as the original, but it still tastes very good and has significantly fewer calories (less than 200) and less fat (only 1 gram saturated) than its traditional deli counterpart. You can toast the bread for a crisper base.

Serving Suggestions: Prepare a white potato salad or, even better, a sweet potato salad, accented with slivers of sun-dried tomatoes and dressed with an eggless soy mayonnaise mixed with a little Dijon mustard.

MAKES 4 OPEN-FACED SANDWICHES
Prep: 5 minutes / Cook: about 10 minutes

    4 slices rye or whole-grain bread
    4 tablespoons Thousand Island Dressing (page 138)
    8 slices meatless bacon strips, cooked according to package directions, or 4 slices soy
        Canadian bacon slices
    1 cup refrigerated sauerkraut, rinsed and well drained
    4 thin slices or 1 cup shredded (about 4 ounces) Swiss-style soy cheese

1. Heat oven to 375°F.

2. Place bread slices on a baking sheet. Spread each slice with 1 tablespoon dressing, then top with 2 bacon slices, $\frac{1}{4}$ cup sauerkraut, and 1 slice cheese.

3. Bake until heated through and cheese is melted, about 10 minutes. Serve immediately.

Sloppy Joes

This sloppy Joe mixture gets even tastier the second and third day. Ketchup, once considered a vegetable by some, is a source of lycopene, along with the canned tomatoes, and the soy "beef" provides a hit of isoflavones.

Serving Suggestions: You can omit the buns and serve the sloppy Joe mixture over regular brown rice or brown basmati rice. Accompany with Homemade Tortilla Chips (page 55) and a green salad topped with shredded carrot.

MAKES 6 SERVINGS (ABOUT 4 CUPS)
Prep: 10 minutes / Cook: 20 minutes

  1 teaspoon olive oil
  1 sweet white onion such as Vidalia, finely chopped
  1 red bell pepper, cored, seeded, and chopped
  1 package (14 ounces) ground beef–style soy
  1 clove garlic, finely chopped
  2 teaspoons chili powder
  $\frac{1}{4}$ teaspoon salt
  $\frac{2}{3}$ cup ketchup
  $\frac{1}{4}$ to $\frac{1}{3}$ cup red wine vinegar, to taste
  2 tablespoons dark brown sugar
  1 tablespoon Worcestershire sauce
  1 can (32 ounces) whole tomatoes, drained and chopped
  6 whole-wheat or other whole-grain soft rolls or buns, split and toasted if desired

1. In a large nonstick skillet, heat oil over medium heat. Add onion and bell pepper and cook, stirring occasionally, until crisp-tender, about 5 minutes.
2. Crumble the soy beef into the skillet. Stir in garlic, chili powder, and salt, and cook, stirring occasionally and breaking up soy crumbles, until vegetables are tender, about 4 minutes.
3. Meanwhile, in a small bowl, stir together ketchup, vinegar, sugar, and Worcestershire.
4. Add tomatoes and ketchup mixture to the skillet and stir to combine. Gently simmer for 10 minutes, stirring occasionally and breaking up tomatoes.
5. Serve sloppy Joe mixture over rolls.

Make-Ahead Tip: Sloppy Joe mixture can be refrigerated for up to three days.

Chili Dog on a Bun

Here's an American favorite translated into a soy-based version with only 1 gram of saturated fat.

Serving Suggestions: To continue the theme, try a potato salad or coleslaw made with an eggless soy mayonnaise, along with flavored Homemade Tortilla Chips (page 55) or store-bought reduced-fat chips for the final touch.

MAKES 1 SERVING
Prep: 5 minutes

> 1 jumbo meatless soy frankfurter
> 1 whole-grain hot dog bun, lightly toasted or steamed until soft and moist
> $\frac{1}{4}$ cup Chili con Soy (page 153)

1. Cook frankfurter using your favorite method—grilled, broiled, boiled—according to package directions.
2. Place hot dog in warm bun. Top with hot chili and serve.

Grilled Sausage and Pepper Hero

For this pizza parlor favorite, instead of grilling the ingredients, you can broil or pan-fry them in olive oil in a nonstick skillet and then toast the bread separately. The cooking times are approximately the same, regardless of cooking method. Lycopene from the tomato sauce and soy in the sausage are the nutritional pluses here, as are the antioxidants in the bell pepper.

Serving Suggestions: For pizza-style sandwiches, use grilled or toasted whole-wheat pocketless pitas in place of buns. A bowl of crispy vegetable chips is a good go-with.

MAKES 4 HEROES
Prep: 10 minutes / Cook: 8 minutes

2 cups Homemade All-Purpose Tomato Sauce (page 259), or bottled meatless marinara sauce

$\frac{1}{4}$ teaspoon crushed red pepper flakes

4 whole-grain hot dog–style rolls, split lengthwise and opened like a book

1 tablespoon olive oil

1 large onion, thickly sliced

2 green, red, yellow, or orange bell peppers, or a combination, cored, seeded, and cut lengthwise into $\frac{1}{2}$-inch-thick slices

1 package (8 ounces) Italian-style soy sausage links, each link split lengthwise

$\frac{1}{2}$ cup shredded mozzarella-style soy cheese (optional)

1. Heat the outdoor grill, indoor nonstick covered grill pan, or broiler. Meanwhile, in a large saucepan, heat tomato sauce and pepper flakes to a simmer. Keep warm.

2. Brush the cut sides of the rolls evenly with olive oil. Grill until lightly toasted, about 2 minutes. Keep warm.

3. Grill or broil onion slices and peppers until crisp-tender and charred, turning over, about 4 minutes. Add to sauce in pan and gently toss.

4. Grill or broil sausages until heated through, about $1\frac{1}{2}$ minutes.

5. Place open rolls on serving plates. Top with sausages. Spoon vegetables and sauce evenly over. Top with cheese, if using, and serve at once.

Chicken Parmesan Melt

Lunch, supper, or a snack—this is satisfying at any meal. In a pinch, you can use a bottled meatless marinara sauce; the sauce is still full of lycopene. And of course, the chicken is not really chicken, but a soy substitute, providing isoflavones. Melts are high in calories but low in saturated fat, so save them for a day when you expect the rest of your calorie intake to be low.

Serving Suggestions: Toss blanched broccoli and bottled roasted red pepper, cut into strips, with a red-wine vinegar and olive oil dressing.

MAKES 4 OPEN-FACED SANDWICHES
Prep: 10 minutes / Cook: 8 minutes

> 1 tablespoon olive oil
>
> 4 frozen chicken-style vegetarian patties
>
> 2 tablespoons grated Parmesan-style soy cheese
>
> 1½ cups Homemade All-Purpose Tomato Sauce (page 259), or bottled meatless marinara sauce
>
> ½ cup (2 ounces) shredded mozzarella-style soy cheese
>
> 2 large (sandwich-size) whole-grain English muffins, split

1. In a large nonstick skillet, heat oil over medium heat. Add patties and cook for 3 minutes. Turn patties over and sprinkle them evenly with Parmesan-style cheese.

2. Add sauce to the skillet and lower heat. Cover and simmer for 3 minutes. Top patties with mozzarella. Cover the skillet again and cook until mozzarella is melted, about 2 minutes.

3. Meanwhile, toast muffins. Place muffin halves on serving plates. Top with patties, spoon on sauce, and serve.

Salmon Salad Sandwich with Red Bell Pepper

Many canned brands of salmon use wild salmon, which is thought by some to be healthier for our diets rather than the more available farm-raised, which may have higher levels of PCBs and mercury (page 189). This recipe also works well with canned tuna (use the firm kind packed in water), but the easily chewed bones in the salmon add a little extra calcium.

Serving Suggestions: Accompany the sandwich with Three-Bean Salad with Edamame (page 129), or serve the salmon salad on its own without the bread as a luncheon or snack plate, arranged with some dark leafy greens and tomato.

MAKES 4 SANDWICHES

Prep: 15 minutes

> 1 can (14.75 ounces) salmon, drained
>
> 4 scallions, trimmed and finely chopped
>
> I medium-size carrot, peeled, trimmed, and shredded
>
> $\frac{1}{2}$ small red bell pepper, cored, seeded, and finely chopped
>
> $\frac{1}{4}$ teaspoon salt
>
> $\frac{1}{4}$ teaspoon black pepper
>
> 3 tablespoons eggless soy-based mayonnaise
>
> 8 slices whole-wheat or other whole-grain bread, toasted if you want
>
> 8 dark green lettuce leaves
>
> 4 tomato slices
>
> 4 large pieces bottled roasted red pepper, drained (optional)

1. In a small bowl, break salmon into small pieces. Stir in scallions, carrot, bell pepper, salt, pepper, and mayonnaise until evenly blended.

2. Make four sandwiches, dividing the salad equally among bread slices and garnishing with lettuce, tomato, and roasted red pepper, if using.

Make-Ahead Tip: Salmon salad can be refrigerated for up to three days.

Variation: Broccoli: Briefly steam or microwave $\frac{1}{2}$ cup of coarsely chopped broccoli florets until firm-tender. Rinse under cold running water to stop the cooking, and drain well. Add to salmon mixture.

Tuna Fish Salad Sandwich with Scallion and Pickled Ginger

The pickled ginger, which comes in jars and can be found in the Asian section of your supermarket, adds a pleasantly unexpected sweet pungency to the salad. For a very special tuna salad, grill or broil 12 ounces of fresh tuna. Remove and discard the skin, break the meat up into small pieces, and use it as the base for the sandwich filler below. Tuna is a cold-water fish that has a high percentage of omega-3s. You can also substitute canned salmon for the tuna.

Serving Suggestions: For a sharply flavored accompaniment, toss together Spicy Cabbage Salad with Cider Vinegar (page 120), or serve the tuna salad as is on a bed of dark leafy greens with bottled roasted red peppers as a garnish.

MAKES 4 SANDWICHES

Prep: 10 minutes

> 1 can (12 ounces) solid white tuna packed in water, drained
>
> 2 scallions, trimmed and finely chopped
>
> 1 tablespoon finely chopped pickled ginger
>
> 2 tablespoons eggless soy-based mayonnaise
>
> $\frac{1}{4}$ teaspoon salt
>
> $\frac{1}{4}$ teaspoon black pepper
>
> Hot red pepper sauce, to taste (optional)
>
> 8 slices whole-wheat or other whole-grain bread, toasted if you want
>
> 8 dark green lettuce leaves
>
> 4 tomato slices
>
> 4 large pieces bottled roasted red pepper, drained (optional)

1. In a small bowl, break up tuna with fork. Add scallion, pickled ginger, mayonnaise, salt, pepper, and hot pepper sauce if using, and mix together with fork.
2. Make four sandwiches with the bread, dividing the salad equally among them, and garnishing with lettuce, tomato, and roasted red pepper, if using.

Make-Ahead Tip: Salad can be refrigerated for up to three days.

Black Bean and Vegetable Tostada with Avocado and Lime

This is a light meal in itself, easily assembled by anyone in the family. It also makes a delicious impromptu snack. The beans and the corn provide complementary protein, and avocado, rich in omega–3 fatty acids, is thought to have prostate cancer–fighting properties. For more heat, the fresh chile can be replaced with a canned chipotle chile in adobo or with a pickled jalapeño.

Serving Suggestions: Shredded carrots or shredded romaine lettuce, tossed with a mustard-honey vinaigrette, makes an easy crunchy side salad. Or toss slivered jicama and radishes with a little freshly squeezed lime juice.

MAKES 6 SERVINGS
Prep: 15 minutes / Cook: about 10 minutes

> Six 6-inch corn tortillas, low-fat if available
> Nonstick olive oil cooking spray
> 1 can (15 ounces) black beans, drained and rinsed
> 1 can (11 ounces) canned corn kernels, drained and rinsed
> 1 small tomato, cored and chopped
> 2 tablespoons finely chopped red onion
> 1 small fresh jalapeño, seeded and finely chopped
> 2 tablespoons chopped fresh cilantro
> 1 tablespoon freshly squeezed lime juice
> $\frac{1}{2}$ teaspoon salt
> $\frac{1}{8}$ to $\frac{1}{4}$ teaspoon hot red pepper sauce
> 1 small ripe avocado, pitted, peeled, and chopped

1. Heat oven to 450°F. Coat both sides of tortillas with cooking spray. Place tortillas in single layer on baking sheets.

2. Bake tortillas until lightly browned and crisp, 6 to 10 minutes, flipping them over halfway through. Transfer tortillas to a wire rack and let cool.

3. In a large bowl, gently stir together black beans, corn kernels, tomato, onion, jalapeño, cilantro, lime juice, salt, and pepper sauce to taste. Gently fold in avocado. Spoon $\frac{1}{2}$ cup onto each tortilla and serve.

Make-Ahead Tip: The filling, without the avocado, can be made a day ahead and refrigerated.

Corn Tortilla Wrap with Sun-Dried Tomato Pesto and Jack Cheese

This is one of those sandwiches that can be quickly thrown together when you want a no-effort lunch or a substantial snack—no saturated fat and only about 100 calories.

Serving Suggestions: Accompany with a chicory and Belgian endive salad or a shredded spinach salad with orange segments.

MAKES 4 SANDWICHES
Prep: 5 minutes / Cook: 30 seconds

> Four 6-inch corn tortillas, low-fat if available
> $\frac{1}{4}$ cup bottled sun-dried tomato pesto
> 4 slices Monterey jack–style, mozzarella-style, or Swiss-style soy cheese

Over each tortilla, spread 1 tablespoon pesto. Top with cheese and roll up. Microwave or broil until cheese melts, about 30 seconds.

Ham and Herbed Cheese Roll-Up

Ready in less than ten minutes! Ideal for a quick lunch or snack, or even for evening television watching. The ham is made from soy, so isoflavones are part of the deal.

Serving Suggestions: When you steam vegetables for dinner, always try to make extra. Then when you prepare a quick sandwich, you can create an instant salad accompaniment from leftover broccoli, cauliflower, green beans, snow peas, or whatever it is you have in the refrigerator, tossing them with Balsamic Vinaigrette (page 141).

MAKES 2 SANDWICHES
Prep: 5 minutes / Cook: 1 minute

> 1 spinach or sun-dried tomato–flavored 8-inch tortilla
> 2 tablespoons Herbed Cheese Spread with Sun-Dried Tomatoes (page 48)
> 1 Romaine, curly, or Boston lettuce leaf
> 2 country ham–style soy slices

1. Heat tortilla, according to package directions.

2. Spread warm tortilla with cheese. Top with lettuce leaf. Overlap ham-style slices on one side of tortilla. Gently roll up tortilla, cut in half, and serve.

Turkey and Bacon Sandwich with Avocado-Chipotle Mayonnaise

This is a delicious sandwich, rich in soy. And recent studies suggest that a particular antioxidant in avocados may inhibit the growth of prostate cancer.

Serving Suggestions: Toss seedless orange segments with a splash of balsamic vinegar and arrange over baby spinach leaves for a cooling salad accompaniment. To create a more substantial lunch or light supper, serve with small bowls of Garden Gazpacho with Edamame (page 112), or Tomato and Red Bell Pepper Soup with Basil (page 100).

MAKES 4 SANDWICHES.

Prep: 15 minutes / Cook: about 3 minutes

1 ripe avocado

$\frac{1}{2}$ cup Chipotle Mayonnaise (page 264)

1 tablespoon freshly squeezed lime juice

8 slices meatless soy bacon

8 slices whole-wheat bread, toasted

1 tomato, cored and thinly sliced

12 slices (6-ounce package) turkey-style soy slices

1. Halve and seed avocado. Scoop flesh into a small bowl and mash. Stir in mayonnaise and lime juice.

2. Cook soy bacon according to package directions.

3. Spread 4 slices of toast each with 2 tablespoons mayonnaise. For each sandwich, layer on 2 bacon slices, tomato, 3 turkey slices, and final slice of bread. Cut in half and serve.

Sausage and Mozzarella Stuffed Bread

If you're having some friends in to watch a football game or political debate on TV, serve this as a party loaf. When you make this recipe, allow enough time for the dough to thaw and rise. And it's easy to double the recipe to make two loaves, so you can have a spare one stored in the freezer. Look for the bread dough in the freezer section of your supermarket. There's negligible saturated fat in the loaf, while each slice packs a walloping 20 grams of protein.

Serving Suggestions: For a pleasantly assertive salad, toss together arugula and red leaf lettuce with a Balsamic Vinaigrette (page 141). The sausage mixture, without the cheese, doubles as a pasta sauce when thinned with a couple tablespoons of pasta cooking water or vegetable broth.

MAKES 16 SLICES
Prep: 20 minutes / Cook: 40 minutes

> 1 loaf (about 1 pound) frozen bread dough
> Nonstick olive oil cooking spray
> 1 tablespoon olive oil
> 1 sweet onion such as Vidalia, halved and thinly sliced crosswise
> 1 red bell pepper, cored, seeded, and cut into thin strips
> 3 cloves garlic, finely chopped
> 1 package (14 ounces) Italian-style sweet or hot soy sausage links, sliced into $\frac{1}{4}$-inch-thick pieces
> 1 cup Homemade All-Purpose Tomato Sauce (page 259) or bottled meatless marinara sauce
> 1 cup (4 ounces) shredded mozzarella-style soy cheese
> Liquid egg substitute equal to 1 egg

1. Thaw frozen bread dough, according to package directions. Let rise and punch down.
2. Heat oven to 400°F. Lightly coat a large baking sheet with cooking spray.
3. In a large nonstick skillet, heat oil over medium heat. Add onion and bell pepper and cook, stirring occasionally, until softened, about 6 minutes. Add garlic and cook for 1 minute. Stir in sausage and heat through, about 3 minutes, being careful not to overcook sausage. Stir in tomato sauce and cheese, and cook, stirring, for 1 minute. Remove from heat.

4. On a lightly floured work surface, roll out dough to a 12 x 8-inch rectangle. Spoon sausage filling lengthwise down the center of the dough, leaving a 1-inch border at the ends. Fold the long sides over filling, pinching seam to seal. Fold the short ends over and pinch to seal. Place loaf, seam side down, on the prepared baking sheet. Brush loaf with egg substitute.

5. Bake until loaf is golden brown and sounds firm when rapped with knuckles, about 30 minutes. Transfer to a wire rack and let cool. Slice with a serrated knife and serve warm or at room temperature.

Make-Ahead Tip: The baked loaf can be refrigerated for up to three days or frozen for up to a month. Serve at room temperature or rewarm in a microwave or in a conventional oven at 350°F.

Chickpea Burger with Almonds and Ginger

Store-bought veggie burgers are good to have on hand for an instant lunch, but with homemade you know exactly what's in them. Although you could skip the fresh ginger, it really does make a big difference in the flavor. Each burger delivers 6 grams of fiber.

Serving Suggestions: For a sandwich, use whole-wheat toast or a whole-wheat pita pocket or English muffin. Top the patties with bottled chutney, bottled roasted red bell pepper, or fresh tomato and lettuce. For dinner, serve one or two patties on their own with brown basmati rice and steamed broccoli or carrots, sprinkled with chopped parsley or cilantro.

MAKES 4 BURGERS
Prep: 15 minutes / Cook: 10 minutes

   1 can (15 ounces) chickpeas, drained and rinsed
   4 scallions, trimmed and cut into short lengths
   2 slices whole-wheat bread, torn into pieces
   $\frac{1}{3}$ cup almonds
   $\frac{3}{4}$ teaspoon ground cumin
   2 tablespoons peeled, chopped fresh ginger
   $\frac{1}{2}$ teaspoon salt
   $\frac{1}{4}$ teaspoon black pepper
   1 large egg white
   Nonstick olive oil cooking spray

1. In a food processor, combine chickpeas, scallions, bread, almonds, cumin, ginger, salt, and pepper. Pulse until coarsely chopped. Remove half the mixture to a bowl.
2. Add egg white to the mixture remaining in the processor. Process until smooth. Add to the mixture in the bowl and blend together with spoon. Make four equal patties, about $\frac{3}{4}$ inch thick.
3. Coat a large nonstick skillet with cooking spray, and heat over medium-high heat. Add burgers and cook until browned and heated through, 3 to 5 minutes a side.

Make-Ahead Tip: Uncooked burgers can be refrigerated for up to a day or frozen for up to a month.

Sweet Potato Burger with Kale and Black-Eyed Peas

Hidden away in this burger are a whole host of nutrient- and antioxidant-rich ingredients: kale, sweet potatoes, black-eyed peas, garlic, and tofu. These patties generate only 150 calories, with 5 grams of fiber and no saturated fat.

Serving Suggestions: Serve in whole-wheat pita bread or on whole-grain buns or bread, toasted if you like, spread with BBQ sauce or mustard, and topped with sliced tomato and lettuce for the royal treatment. On their own, the patties are delicious accompanied with soy-milk mashed potatoes enlivened with Dijon mustard and horseradish, and Scalloped Corn with Sun-Dried Tomatoes (p. 248).

MAKES 8 BURGERS
Prep: 15 minutes / Refrigerate: 30 minutes / Cook: 35 minutes

> 2 tablespoons olive oil
>
> 1 cup (about 1 bunch) chopped scallions
>
> 1 large red bell pepper, cored, seeded, and coarsely chopped
>
> $\frac{1}{2}$ small bunch (6 ounces) kale, stemmed and chopped
>
> 3 large cloves garlic, finely chopped
>
> 2 teaspoons Cajun seasoning
>
> 2 small (1 pound) sweet potatoes, peeled and shredded
>
> 1 can (15 ounces) black-eyed peas, drained and rinsed
>
> 4 ounces firm tofu, drained and blotted dry with paper towels
>
> $\frac{1}{2}$ teaspoon salt
>
> Cornmeal, for coating

1. In a large nonstick skillet, heat 1 tablespoon of the oil over medium heat. Add scallions and cook, stirring occasionally, until softened, about 2 minutes. Add bell pepper and cook until crisp-tender, about 5 minutes. Stir in kale, garlic, and Cajun seasoning and cook, stirring frequently, until kale wilts, about 4 minutes. Add sweet potatoes and cook, stirring occasionally, until they soften, about 10 minutes. Remove from heat.

2. In a large bowl, mash together black-eyed peas and tofu with potato masher. Stir in sweet potato mixture and salt until well blended. Refrigerate until cool enough to handle, about 30 minutes.

3. Spread cornmeal out on piece of waxed paper. Shape mixture into eight patties, about

$3\frac{1}{2}$ inches in diameter, using about $\frac{1}{2}$ cup for each. Sprinkle both sides lightly with corn-meal. (Handle patties carefully as they are fragile.)

4. Wipe out the skillet and heat half of the remaining oil over medium-high heat. Add four patties, reduce heat to medium, and cook until hot and browned, about 5 minutes per side. Remove to a plate and keep warm. Repeat with remaining oil and patties.

Make-Ahead Tip: Uncooked patties can be refrigerated for up to two days or frozen for up to a month.

Red Bean and Brazil Nut Burger with Rosemary

The Brazil nuts add richness as well as selenium, and the edamame and red beans are the sources of protein. If you can find ripe avocados, use them as a garnish. There is also a hefty 12 grams of fiber in each burger.

Serving Suggestions: Coleslaw made with an eggless soy-based mayonnaise, or a tomato salad, is a good side. Or, if serving the burger bunless, top it with Lemon-Mustard Sauce with Horseradish (page 257) and fill out the plate with mashed sweet potatoes.

MAKES 4 BURGERS

Prep: 15 minutes / Refrigerate: 30 minutes / Cook: 8 minutes

1 cup frozen shelled and blanched edamame

$\frac{2}{3}$ cup unsalted Brazil nuts

1 slice whole-wheat bread, torn into pieces

2 scallions, trimmed and cut into 1-inch pieces

1 cup canned small red beans, drained and rinsed

1 large egg white or liquid egg substitute equal to 1 egg

$\frac{1}{4}$ cup fresh parsley leaves, chopped

1 teaspoon dried rosemary, crushed

$\frac{1}{4}$ teaspoon salt

$\frac{1}{4}$ teaspoon black pepper

1 tablespoon olive oil

4 whole-wheat hamburger buns, toasted

4 slices tomato

4 dark-green lettuce leaves

1 ripe avocado, halved, peeled, pitted, and cut into thin slices (optional)

1. Cook edamame according to the package directions. Drain well.

2. In a food processor, chop nuts until medium-fine. Transfer to a plate and set aside. In the processor, finely crumb bread, about 1 minute. Add to nuts.

3. Add scallions and edamame to processor, and pulse together until chopped. Add beans, egg white, parsley, rosemary, salt, and pepper. Process until combined. Add reserved nuts and bread crumbs and pulse together just until blended. Form mixture into four $3\frac{1}{2}$ -inch patties, about $\frac{1}{2}$ inch thick. Cover and refrigerate for at least 30 minutes to firm.

4. In a large nonstick skillet, heat oil over medium-low heat. Add patties and cook until golden brown, 3 to 4 minutes on each side. Serve on buns with tomato, lettuce, and avocado if using.

Make-Ahead Tip: Uncooked patties can be made a day ahead and refrigerated, or frozen for up to one month.

CHAPTER IV

SOUPS

SOUPS CAN BE ANYTHING YOU WANT them to be, as they have been since people began to cook. They serve well as a snack, a first course, an appetizer, or a main dish, depending on what you put in them. I even sometimes sip a mugful of homemade tomato soup or—in the summer—chilled cantaloupe soup as I drive to my next appointment.

Because soups are so versatile and adaptable, it is easy to transform favorite recipes as well as create new ones that conform to a prostate-savvy diet, and at the same time satisfy the whole family's appetite. Knowing a few easy tricks will help you accomplish this. Meat-based stocks can be replaced with a homemade (page 101) or store-bought vegetable broth, and meat or chicken removed in favor of grains and/or legumes, or soybeans and tofu, combined with a cornucopia of vegetables for an abundance of antioxidants. Take the heavy cream out of cream soups, but keep the creamy texture by stirring in pureed vegetables or beans, as in Cream of Broccoli-Carrot Soup (page 96).

A variety of different vegetable broths are available in supermarkets. The Imagine brand is one of my favorites.

In this chapter recipes reflect a variety of ethnic influences: Portuguese-inspired White Bean and Kale Soup with Pasta (page 102), Thai Noodle Soup with Vegetables and Edamame (page 98), Tortilla Soup with Serrano Chile (page 103), and Corn and Edamame Chowder with Sweet Potato (page 106).

Roasted Butternut Squash Soup with Curry and Coconut

Just a hint of curry powder and coconut milk give this winter warmer its subtly sweet flavor. And the orange-colored squash is an excellent source of antioxidants. Roasting the squash adds to the cooking time, but it also enhances the flavor of the soup. To speed up the preparation process, but with a different taste result, you can substitute $1\frac{1}{4}$ cups canned solid-pack pumpkin puree for the roasted squash.

Although coconut milk does contain a high percentage of fat, a little goes a long way, and it contributes such great flavor to a dish that it's tasty fun to use it in recipes from time to time. Coconut milk also comes in "lite" or reduced-fat versions—compare them to regular coconut milk to see which you prefer, since flavors can be different, depending on the brand.

Serving Suggestions: For an extra garnish, spoon a little plain soy yogurt over the top. Accompany the soup with Homemade Pita Chips (page 53) and a pungent watercress and Belgian endive salad, tossed with white-wine vinegar dressing and flavored with a pinch of ground cumin.

MAKES 6 SERVINGS
Prep: 20 minutes / Cook: 45 minutes

Nonstick olive oil cooking spray

1 medium-size ($1\frac{1}{2}$ pounds) butternut or acorn squash, halved lengthwise and seeded

1 teaspoon olive oil

1 large onion, finely chopped

2 cloves garlic, finely chopped

1 teaspoon salt

$\frac{1}{2}$ teaspoon curry powder

1 medium-size potato (Yukon gold if available), peeled and chopped

1 large carrot, trimmed, peeled, and finely chopped

4 cups vegetable broth, homemade (page 101) or store-bought, or water

$\frac{1}{2}$ cup canned regular or "lite" coconut milk

Chopped fresh cilantro, for garnish (optional)

1. Heat oven to 400°F. Line a baking pan with aluminum foil. Lightly coat foil with cooking spray. Place squash halves, cut-side down, on foil.

2. Roast squash until very tender, about 45 minutes.

3. Meanwhile, in a large nonstick saucepan, heat oil over medium heat. Add onion and cook, stirring occasionally, until softened, about 5 minutes. Add garlic, $\frac{1}{2}$ teaspoon of the salt, and curry powder, and cook for 1 minute longer.

4. Add potato, carrot, and broth. Bring to a boil. Reduce heat to low and simmer, uncovered, until vegetables are very tender, about 15 minutes. Remove from heat and let cool slightly.

5. When squash is tender, carefully remove skin. Working in batches if necessary, and giving ingredients time to cool enough for pureeing, combine soup mixture, squash, and coconut milk in a food processor or blender. Whirl until almost smooth. Reheat gently before serving. Garnish with cilantro, if using.

Make-Ahead Tip: Soup can be refrigerated for up to two days or frozen for up to a month. The squash can be roasted a day ahead and refrigerated.

Cream of Broccoli-Carrot Soup

The broccoli and carrots deliver a healthy dose of antioxidants, the beans and soy milk combine to provide nonanimal sources of protein, and all the ingredients together add up to 9 grams of fiber per serving. The cooking trick that creates the impression of rich creaminess is pureeing the cannellini beans.

Serving Suggestions: Pair with a green salad topped with thinly sliced apple tossed with lemon juice, and garnished with chopped, toasted Brazil nuts. For a heartier meal, add a roasted vegetable sandwich.

MAKES 4 SERVINGS
Prep: 15 minutes / Cook: 20 minutes

1 tablespoon olive oil

1 sweet onion such as Vidalia, coarsely chopped

1 small head broccoli, stems peeled, and both crown and stems coarsely chopped

2 carrots, trimmed, peeled, and coarsely chopped

4 cups vegetable broth, homemade (page 101) or store-bought

1 can (15 ounces) cannellini beans, drained and rinsed

About 1 cup unsweetened soy milk

$\frac{1}{2}$ teaspoon dried dill

$\frac{1}{4}$ teaspoon salt

$\frac{1}{8}$ teaspoon black pepper

1. In a large nonstick saucepan, heat oil over medium heat. Add onion and cook, stirring occasionally, until softened, about 5 minutes. Add broccoli, carrots, and vegetable broth. Simmer, covered, until broccoli is just tender, 8 to 10 minutes. Set aside until cool enough to puree.

2. In a food processor, working in batches if necessary, puree broccoli and carrots along with a little of the cooking liquid. Stir back into remaining cooking liquid in saucepan.

3. In the processor, puree cannellini beans with about $\frac{1}{4}$ cup of the soy milk. Stir into broccoli mixture.

4. Gradually stir in enough of the remaining soy milk for desired consistency. Stir in dill, salt, and pepper and simmer for 5 minutes to blend flavors.

Make-Ahead Tip: Soup can be refrigerated for up to two days.

Curried Pumpkin Soup with Cauliflower

This soup is a treasure trove of antioxidants, derived from the cauliflower, a cruciferous vegetable, and the pumpkin puree, rich in beta-carotene.

Serving Suggestions: For a garnish, spoon plain soy yogurt on top and dollop with a little chutney.

MAKES 6 SERVINGS
Prep: 10 minutes / Cook: 35 minutes

> 2 tablespoons olive oil
> 2 cups coarsely chopped, trimmed cauliflower
> 1 sweet onion such as Vidalia, coarsely chopped
> 1 tablespoon curry powder
> 4 cups vegetable broth, homemade (page 101) or store-bought
> 1 can (16 ounces) solid-pack pumpkin puree (not pie filling)
> $\frac{3}{4}$ teaspoon salt

1. In a large nonstick saucepan, heat oil over medium heat. Add cauliflower and cook, stirring occasionally, until crisp-tender, about 5 minutes. Remove cauliflower to a bowl.

2. Add onion and curry powder to the saucepan and cook, stirring occasionally, until onion is softened, about 5 minutes. Add 2 cups of the broth and bring to a boil. Lower heat, cover, and simmer for 15 minutes. Let cool slightly.

3. Working in batches, puree the onion mixture in a blender or small food processor until smooth. Return the mixture to the saucepan.

4. Stir in the remaining 2 cups broth, pumpkin, salt, and cauliflower. Bring to a boil. Then lower heat, cover, and simmer until cauliflower is tender, about 10 minutes.

Make-Ahead Tip: Soup can be refrigerated for up to three days.

Thai Noodle Soup with Vegetables and Edamame

Bright flavors are the hallmark of this Asian-seasoned soup, which is also a tasty introduction to rice noodles, as well as protein-rich edamame. You can easily control the level of heat with the pepper sauce—and for more complex heat, you can add a chopped, seeded, fresh serrano chile along with the mushrooms in step 2. For best flavor, serve soon after making.

Serving Suggestions: This is a meal in itself, but sliced cucumbers tossed with a little rice vinegar would be a heat-tempering addition on the side. Or try serving the soup as a first course before broiled fish.

MAKES 4 SERVINGS

Prep: 25 minutes / Cook: 25 minutes

2 ounces dried rice noodles or fettuccine

1 lime

2 teaspoons olive oil

4 ounces white button mushrooms, cleaned, tough stems discarded, and sliced (about 2 cups)

2 medium-size carrots, trimmed, peeled, and thinly sliced

$\frac{1}{2}$ red bell pepper, cored, seeded, and thinly sliced into 2-inch lengths

2 cloves garlic, finely chopped

$1\frac{3}{4}$ cups vegetable broth, homemade (page 101) or store-bought

$\frac{1}{2}$ cup canned regular or "lite" coconut milk

2 teaspoons regular or reduced-sodium soy sauce

2 teaspoons peeled, finely chopped fresh ginger

$1\frac{1}{2}$ teaspoons honey

$\frac{1}{2}$ teaspoon anchovy paste, or 1 teaspoon Thai or Vietnamese fish sauce (optional; omit the salt if using)

1–2 teaspoons jalapeño pepper sauce or other hot sauce

1 cup frozen shelled and blanched edamame

4 scallions, trimmed and sliced (about $\frac{1}{2}$ cup)

$\frac{1}{4}$ teaspoon salt

$\frac{1}{4}$ cup fresh cilantro leaves, coarsely chopped (optional)

1. Cook noodles according to package directions. Drain well and set aside. Grate 1 teaspoon lime zest from lime and squeeze 1½ teaspoons juice and set both aside.

2. In a wok or large skillet, heat oil over medium-high heat. Add mushrooms, carrots, bell pepper, and garlic and cook, stirring, until softened, about 5 minutes. Add broth, coconut milk, soy sauce, ginger, honey, and anchovy paste, if using, and pepper sauce to taste. Bring to a simmer. Stir in edamame, scallions, and salt if not using the anchovy paste or fish sauce, and simmer until edamame are just tender, about 3 minutes.

3. Stir in cooked noodles, and lime juice and zest, and cook until heated through, about 1 minute. Serve in shallow bowls, topping with cilantro, if using.

Make-Ahead Tip: Best served right after making, but can be refrigerated for up to a day.

Tomato and Red Bell Pepper Soup with Basil

Although canned tomatoes work just fine in this soup, it's hard to beat the flavor of ripe late-summer tomatoes. The tomatoes and the red bell pepper combine for a bonanza of antioxidants, and the olive oil makes the lycopene in the tomatoes more bio-available. Although this recipe is not as quick as many others in this book, the initial cooking down of the tomatoes and bell peppers really concentrates the flavor. For an extra protein boost, add 1 cup frozen shelled and blanched edamame in step 3 and simmer for 5 minutes.

Serving Suggestions: Keep it simple—whole-grain crackers, crusty whole-grain bread, little Homemade Crostini (page 56), or Homemade Pita Chips (page 53) and, for a salad, spinach and arugula.

MAKES 4 SERVINGS

Prep: 15 minutes / Cook: about 1 hour

> 1 tablespoon olive oil
>
> 1 large yellow onion, halved and sliced crosswise
>
> 4 tomatoes (about 2 pounds), cored, peeled, seeded, and chopped, or 1 can (28 ounces) peeled whole tomatoes, seeded and chopped
>
> 2 red bell peppers, cored, seeded, and chopped
>
> 1 teaspoon dried basil
>
> $\frac{1}{2}$ teaspoon salt
>
> $\frac{1}{4}$ teaspoon black pepper
>
> 3 cups vegetable broth, homemade (page 101) or store-bought
>
> $\frac{1}{4}$ cup fresh basil leaves, cut into thin strips as garnish (optional)

1. In a large nonstick saucepan, heat oil over medium heat. Add onion and cook, stirring occasionally, until softened, about 5 minutes. Stir in tomatoes and bell peppers. Reduce heat to medium-low and cook, stirring occasionally, until juices have evaporated, about 30 minutes. Be sure to stir more often at the end to prevent scorching.

2. Stir in dried basil, salt, pepper, and broth. Bring to a boil. Lower heat and simmer, stirring occasionally, to blend flavors, 25 minutes.

3. Place a sieve over a large bowl. Strain the soup through the sieve. In a food processor, working in batches, puree solids. Whisk puree into the liquid in the bowl and return soup to saucepan. Gently reheat. Ladle into bowls and garnish with fresh basil, if using.

Make-Ahead Tip: Soup can be refrigerated up to three days or frozen up to a month.

Basic Vegetable Broth

Good-quality commercially prepared vegetable broths are available, but if you make your own, then you know exactly what's in it and you can control the amount of added salt. For a slight sweetness, add whole cloves or star anise along with the bay leaf—remember to remove these before using the broth.

Serving Suggestions: Use in any of your own recipes that call for chicken or beef broth. For a practically instant soup, warm some of this stock, then add small cubes of firm tofu, Five-Spice Tofu (page 65) or Tofu Snack Triangles with Ginger and Honey (page 64).

MAKES ABOUT 6 CUPS
Prep. 5 minutes / Cook: about 1 hour

> 1 tablespoon olive oil
>
> 1 large sweet onion such as Vidalia, coarsely chopped
>
> 2 stalks celery, coarsely chopped
>
> 2 carrots, trimmed, peeled, and coarsely chopped
>
> 3 cloves garlic, with skins on, crushed with a side of a chef's knife
>
> $\frac{1}{4}$ teaspoon salt
>
> $\frac{1}{4}$ cup coarsely chopped fresh parsley
>
> 1 bay leaf

1. In a large saucepan, heat oil over medium heat. Add onion, celery, carrots, garlic, and salt and cook, covered, stirring occasionally, until slightly softened, about 5 minutes. Add 8 cups water, parsley, and bay leaf. Bring to a boil. Reduce heat to medium-low and simmer, uncovered, for 1 hour.

2. Strain stock through a fine-mesh sieve placed over large bowl. Gently press the solids with a rubber spatula or back of a large spoon to squeeze out juices. Discard solids.

3. Use stock as is, or for a more concentrated flavor, boil to reduce by one quarter to one half.

Make-Ahead Tip: Broth can be refrigerated for up to three days or frozen for up to a month. If you make concentrated stock, for easier storage, pour it into ice cube trays, freeze, then pop out the cubes and store them in a freezer bag in freezer. Several cubes are the beginning of a soup, and two or three can be used for steaming vegetables.

White Bean and Kale Soup with Pasta

The list of benefits found in kale is practically endless: the antioxidants beta-carotene, vitamin C, and vitamin E, and several phytonutrients that are thought to have prostate cancer–fighting properties.

Serving Suggestions: Crispy whole-grain bread sticks and sliced tomatoes sprinkled with black pepper and balsamic vinegar are easy accompaniments.

MAKES 8 SERVINGS

Prep: 15 minutes / Cook: 20 minutes

2 tablespoons olive oil

2 stalks celery, diced

2 medium-size carrots, trimmed, peeled, and sliced $\frac{1}{4}$ inch thick

1 medium-size onion, diced

1 clove garlic, finely chopped

1 can (19 ounces) cannellini beans, drained and rinsed

3 cups vegetable broth, homemade (page 101) or store-bought

$\frac{1}{2}$ teaspoon dried rosemary, crushed

$\frac{1}{2}$ teaspoon salt

$\frac{1}{4}$ teaspoon black pepper

$1\frac{1}{2}$ cups frozen chopped kale, collard greens, or chopped spinach (from 1 pound bag frozen)

$\frac{1}{2}$ cup small shell pasta, cooked according to package directions and drained

Grated Parmesan-style soy cheese, for garnish

1. In a large saucepan or pot, heat oil over medium-high heat. Add celery, carrots, onion, and garlic, and cook, stirring frequently, until softened, about 8 minutes.

2. Add beans, broth, rosemary, salt, and pepper, and heat through, about 5 minutes.

3. Using a slotted spoon, transfer 1 cup beans to a bowl. Mash with a potato masher or fork. Stir back into soup. Add kale. Bring to a boil. Lower heat and simmer until kale is heated through, about 10 minutes.

4. Stir pasta into soup. Sprinkle with cheese and serve.

Make-Ahead Tip: Soup can be refrigerated for up to three days. Since the pasta will absorb liquid as it stands in the soup, you may want to thin it with more vegetable broth.

Tortilla Soup with Serrano Chile

This is a very tasty way to get a lycopene boost—you can use either fresh plum tomatoes or canned whole. The recipe is easily doubled or tripled for a crowd. For extra spicy heat, substitute a canned chipotle chile in adobo for the serrano.

Serving Suggestions: Garnish with finely diced avocado and crushed tortilla chips or shredded Monterey Jack–style soy cheese. Serve as a first course before broiled fish or as lunch or a light supper with an orange and jicama salad.

MAKES 4 SERVINGS
Prep: 10 minutes / Cook: 40 minutes

>   3 tablespoons olive oil
>   Two 6-inch corn tortillas
> $\frac{1}{2}$ small sweet onion such as Vidalia, chopped
>   1 clove garlic, finely chopped
>   1 fresh serrano chile, cored, seeded, and chopped
>   1 teaspoon dried oregano
>   5 plum tomatoes, fresh or canned whole, halved lengthwise
>   4 cups vegetable broth, homemade (page 101) or store-bought
>   2 teaspoons freshly squeezed lime juice
> $\frac{1}{2}$ teaspoon salt
> $\frac{1}{4}$ teaspoon black pepper

1. In a large nonstick skillet, heat 2 tablespoons of the oil over medium-high heat. Add tortillas and fry until crisp, turning them once, about 2 minutes per side. Remove to paper towels and blot dry. Break into crispy pieces.

2. In a large nonstick saucepan, heat the remaining tablespoon oil over medium heat. Add onion and cook, stirring occasionally, until softened and lightly browned, about 4 minutes. Add garlic, chile, and oregano and cook for 1 minute. Stir in tomatoes, tortilla pieces, and broth. Bring to a boil. Lower heat and simmer, uncovered, for 30 minutes.

3. Working in batches if necessary, spoon soup into a food processor. Process until pureed. For a smoother texture, use the back of a rubber spatula or large spoon to force the soup through a fine-mesh sieve or strainer into a large bowl. Stir in lime juice, salt, and pepper. Rewarm if necessary.

Make-Ahead Tip: Soup can be refrigerated for up to two days.

Mexican Corn Stew with Red Beans and Chiles

This is an entire meal and is perfect for a crowd. You need nothing else, except maybe a glass of hearty red wine, which some suggest has prostate cancer-fighting properties. Beans and corn are complementary proteins; the carrots, red bell pepper, and salsa provide lots of antioxidants; and the salsa is a good source of lyocpene. The number of calories is a very sensible 255, and the fiber is significant at 10 grams. You can use all small red beans or half red beans and half canned yellow soybeans for an added bonus of isoflavones.

MAKES 6 SERVINGS

Prep: 15 minutes / Cook: 25 minutes

1 tablespoon olive oil

1 small sweet onion such as Vidalia, chopped

2 cloves garlic, finely chopped

3 carrots, trimmed, peeled, and thinly sliced

2 red bell peppers, cored, seeded, and cut into small dice

1 can (4 ounces) chopped jalapeños

$\frac{1}{2}$ cup bottled salsa

2 cans (15 ounces each) small red beans, drained and rinsed, or 1 can small red beans plus 1 can yellow soybeans, drained and rinsed

3 cups vegetable broth, homemade (page 101) or store-bought

3 cups frozen corn kernels

2 teaspoons ground cumin

2 teaspoons ground coriander

$\frac{1}{2}$ teaspoon salt

1 canned chipotle chile in adobo (optional)

Two 6-inch corn tortillas

Nonstick olive oil cooking spray

$\frac{1}{4}$ cup chopped fresh cilantro

1. In a large nonstick pot, heat oil over medium heat. Add onion and cook, stirring occasionally, until slightly softened, about 3 minutes. Stir in garlic and cook 1 minute. Stir in carrots and bell peppers and cook, stirring occasionally, until softened, about 6 minutes

2. Stir in chiles, salsa, beans, broth, corn, cumin, coriander, salt, and chipotle, if using, and bring to a gentle boil. Lower heat and heat through, about 15 minutes.

3. Meanwhile, stack tortillas and cut into thin strips. Coat a large nonstick skillet with

cooking spray. Heat over medium heat. Add tortilla strips and toast until crispy, tossing frequently, about 5 minutes. Remove from heat.

4. To serve, stir cilantro into stew. Spoon into bowls, top with tortilla strips, and serve.

Make-Ahead Tip: Stew, without cilantro stirred in, can be refrigerated for up to three days or frozen up to a month. Gently reheat and stir in cilantro just before serving. Tortilla strips can be stored in an airtight container at room temperature for up to three days.

Black Bean and Corn Soup with Salsa

Here's a high-fiber soup that goes together in 20 minutes, start to finish.

Serving Suggestions: An arugula and red leaf lettuce salad tossed with Honey-Cilantro Vinaigrette (page 136) is an assertive complement to the strong flavors of the soup.

MAKES 6 SERVINGS
Prep: 5 minutes / Cook: 15 minutes

    1 tablespoon olive oil
    1 medium-size red onion, chopped
    2 cans (15 ounces each) black beans, drained and rinsed
    1 can (11 ounces) corn kernels, drained and rinsed, or $1\frac{1}{2}$ cups frozen corn kernels
    2 cups vegetable broth, homemade (page 101) or store-bought
    1 cup bottled chunky salsa
    1 tablespoon freshly squeezed lime juice (about 1 lime)
    $\frac{1}{2}$ teaspoon salt
    $\frac{1}{8}$ teaspoon black pepper

1. In a large nonstick saucepan, heat oil over medium heat. Add onion and cook, stirring occasionally, until softened, about 5 minutes.

2. Meanwhile, in a small bowl, mash 1 cup of the beans with a potato masher or fork. Stir mashed beans, whole beans, corn, broth, salsa, lime juice, salt, and pepper in with the onion. Simmer, uncovered, until heated through, 10 minutes.

Make-Ahead Tip: Soup can be refrigerated for up to two days.

Corn and Edamame Chowder with Sweet Potato

Cooking the sweet potato in a microwave makes that step very easy—otherwise, just steam it until tender. This chowder is nutrient rich: the antioxidant beta-carotene from the sweet potato, isoflavones as well as nonanimal protein from the soy milk and edamame, and antioxidants from the red bell pepper. For a little extra zip, stir in a canned chipotle chile in adobo, seeded and chopped. The chowder tallies 7 grams of protein and 6 grams of fiber.

Serving Suggestions: Serve with crisp whole-grain flat bread and a sliced radish and cucumber salad.

MAKES 6 SERVINGS

Prep: 25 minutes / Cook: 20 minutes

- 1 large (about 12 ounces) sweet potato, scrubbed
- 2 teaspoons olive oil
- $\frac{1}{2}$ sweet onion such as Vidalia, chopped
- 1 stalk celery, chopped
- 2 cups fresh or frozen corn kernels
- 2 cloves garlic, chopped
- $1\frac{1}{2}$ cups unsweetened soy milk
- 1 cup vegetable broth, homemade (page 101) or store-bought
- $\frac{1}{2}$ red bell pepper, cored, seeded, and chopped
- $\frac{1}{2}$ teaspoon dried thyme
- $\frac{3}{4}$ teaspoon salt
- $\frac{1}{4}$ teaspoon black pepper
- 1 cup frozen shelled and blanched edamame
- 3 tablespoons chopped fresh cilantro or parsley (optional)

1. Pierce sweet potato in several places. Microwave at full power for 5 minutes, or until tender when pierced through center with knife. (Or peel and cut into quarters and steam until tender.) When cool enough to handle, peel and cut sweet potato into $\frac{3}{4}$-inch dice.

2. In a large saucepan, heat oil over medium heat. Add onion and celery and cook, stirring occasionally, until softened, about 6 minutes. Add corn, garlic, and $\frac{1}{2}$ cup of the soy milk. Bring to a simmer and cook for 5 minutes.

3. Remove $\frac{3}{4}$ cup of the vegetables and puree in a blender, along with the remaining soy milk, working in batches if necessary.

4. Add soy milk mixture to saucepan, along with broth, bell pepper, thyme, salt, and pepper. Bring to a simmer and cook for 5 minutes. Stir in edamame and cooked sweet potato, and simmer until vegetables are heated through, about 3 minutes. Stir in cilantro, if using, and serve.

Make-Ahead Tip: Chowder can be refrigerated, without the cilantro, for up to three days. Gently reheat and stir in cilantro just before serving.

Lentil Soup with Kale and Sausage

Here's a hearty cold-weather soup that makes use of some of the best convenience products: canned organic vegetarian lentils, frozen chopped kale, and soy sausage. Everyday, it seems, there are new versions of soy sausage in the supermarket. If the one you're using has a casing, remove and discard it. And in most cases, the 8 ounces called for in the recipe will not use a whole package, so you'll have some left over. Nutritionally the soup delivers 16 grams of protein per serving and 8 grams of fiber, along with only 200 calories and 1 gram saturated fat.

This is the kind of recipe that invites endless variation. You could add frozen corn kernels, frozen peas, a splash of balsamic vinegar, cannellini beans instead of lentils, and on and on.

Serving Suggestions: Crispy bread sticks or a crusty loaf of whole-grain bread—that's it.

MAKES 6 SERVINGS
Prep: 10 minutes / Cook: 30 minutes

  2 teaspoons olive oil

  1 small onion, coarsely chopped

  8 ounces Italian-style or chorizo-style soy sausage

  4 cups vegetable broth, homemade (page 101) or store-bought

  1 package (10 ounces) frozen chopped kale or collard greens, or half of a
    16-ounce bag

  1 can (15 ounces) organic vegetarian lentils

  $\frac{1}{4}$ teaspoon salt

  6 tablespoons grated Parmesan-style soy cheese

1. In a large nonstick saucepan, heat oil over medium heat. Add onion and cook, stirring occasionally, until softened, about 5 minutes.

2. If sausage is wrapped in casing, discard casing. Crumble sausage into the saucepan, and cook, stirring occasionally, for 5 minutes. Add broth and kale. Bring to a boil. Then reduce heat and simmer, covered, for 15 minutes.

3. Stir in lentils and salt and simmer for 5 minutes longer. Ladle into six bowls and sprinkle each with 1 tablespoon Parmesan before serving.

Make-Ahead Tip: Soup can be refrigerated for up to three days, or frozen for up to a month.

Caribbean Sweet Potato Soup with Scallops and Cumin

Based on a recipe in a cookbook I wrote a few years back, *Home Cooking Around the World* (Stewart, Tabori & Chang, 2001), this soup is rich in antioxidants from the sweet potato. The seasoning is spicy-sweet, and some alternative-medicine experts have suggested that an active ingredient in turmeric may have prostate cancer-fighting properties.

Serving Suggestions: A sharp-tasting salad based on watercress or arugula would be a delicious counterpoint to the richness of the soup.

MAKES 4 SERVINGS
Prep: 15 minutes / Cook: 20 minutes

$1\frac{1}{2}$ pounds sweet potatoes, peeled and cubed

3 cups vegetable broth, homemade (page 101) or store-bought, plus additional if needed

4 whole cloves

$\frac{1}{2}$ teaspoon ground turmeric

$\frac{1}{2}$ teaspoon ground cardamom

$\frac{1}{2}$ teaspoon salt

$\frac{1}{8}$ teaspoon cayenne

$\frac{1}{2}$ cup canned regular or "lite" coconut milk

$\frac{1}{2}$ pound sea scallops, halved if large

1 tablespoon freshly squeezed lime juice

Chopped fresh cilantro, for garnish (optional)

1. In a large saucepan, combine sweet potatoes, broth, cloves, and turmeric and bring to a boil. Lower heat and simmer until potatoes are tender, about 15 minutes. Remove cloves and discard. Remove pan from heat and let sit until cool enough to puree.

2. In a food processor, working in batches, puree potatoes with broth. Return to saucepan.

3. Stir in cardamom, salt, cayenne, and coconut milk. Bring to a simmer.

4. Add scallops and continue simmering until cooked through, about 5 minutes, being careful not to overcook scallops. Stir in lime juice. If soup is too thick for your taste, thin with a little more vegetable broth. Garnish with cilantro, if using, and serve.

Make-Ahead Tip: Soup can be prepared up through step 2 a day ahead and refrigerated.

Haddock Chowder with Corn and Tomatoes

The flavor of a fish chowder usually gets better the second day, so try and plan accordingly. Plus, this recipe makes enough for eight servings, so it's perfect for an informal party, summer or winter. Cold-water fish are good deliverers of omega-3 fatty acids. Soy milk replaces the heavy cream usually found in a chowder, while pureeing the cooked potatoes adds the texture of cream. The other tip to keep in mind is to stir the chowder as little as possible after the fish is added so the chunks stay whole. The Canadian-style soy bacon adds a "meaty" background note. For the haddock, you can substitute scrod, cod, or halibut.

Serving Suggestions: A salad of assertive greens, such as arugula, radicchio, endive, and watercress, and a basket of crusty whole-grain bread, would effortlessly round out the menu.

MAKES 8 SERVINGS
Prep: 20 minutes / Cook: 35 minutes

1 tablespoon light olive oil

2 slices Canadian-style soy bacon

1 medium-size onion, finely chopped

1 carrot, trimmed, peeled, and finely chopped

1 pound tomatoes, cored, seeded, and coarsely chopped, or 1 can (14.5 ounces) diced tomatoes, drained

1 pound potatoes (preferably Yukon Gold), scrubbed and cut into small dice

1 bottle (8 ounces) clam juice

1 quart unsweetened soy milk

1 teaspoon dried rosemary

1 teaspoon dried oregano

$\frac{1}{2}$ teaspoon dried thyme

$\frac{1}{4}$ teaspoon salt

$\frac{1}{4}$ teaspoon black pepper

2 cups fresh or frozen corn kernels

$1\frac{1}{4}$ pounds haddock fillets, cut into chunks

Chopped fresh parsley, for garnish

1. In a large nonstick saucepan or pot, heat oil over medium heat. Add bacon and cook for 1 minute. Add onion and carrot, cover pot, and cook over low heat, stirring occasionally, until onion and carrot are softened, about 10 minutes. Add tomatoes and cook, covered, until softened, about 3 minutes.

2. Add potatoes, clam juice, and soy milk. Bring to a gentle boil. Lower heat and simmer, covered, until potatoes are tender, about 8 minutes.

3. Place a colander over a large bowl and pour soup through. In a food processor or blender, working in batches, puree solids, adding a little liquid with each batch. Whisk puree into the drained liquid in the bowl. Return the soup to the saucepan.

4. Add rosemary, oregano, thyme, salt, and pepper. Add corn and fish. Bring to a gentle simmer and cook just until fish begins to flake when prodded with fork, about 10 minutes. Serve warm, garnished with parsley.

Make-Ahead Tip: Chowder can be refrigerated for up to two days. Gently reheat it over low heat, keeping stirring to a minimum so the chunks of fish remain whole.

Garden Gazpacho with Edamame

This is a very thick gazpacho with lots of texture. For a thinner version, stir in a little more tomato juice. The addition of edamame provides an extra shot of soy protein, about 4 grams per serving, as well as disease-fighting isoflavones. And of course there is plenty of lycopene from the tomato. For a slightly "smokier" flavor, substitute half of a bottled roasted red pepper for the fresh bell pepper.

Serving Suggestions: Serve as a first course, a main course with a jicama and radish salad, or even as breakfast eye-opener on a warm summer morning. A coffee mug full makes a great spoonable snack.

MAKES 4 SERVINGS

Prep: 15 minutes

$\frac{3}{4}$ cup frozen shelled and blanched edamame

1 cup tomato juice

1 tomato, cut into eighths

3 ice cubes

One 4-inch-long piece cucumber, peeled, halved lengthwise, seeded, and cut into $\frac{3}{4}$-inch cubes (about $\frac{2}{3}$ cup)

$\frac{1}{2}$ medium-size yellow or red bell pepper, cut into $\frac{3}{4}$-inch cubes (about $\frac{3}{4}$ cup)

2 scallions, trimmed and cut into 1-inch pieces

3 tablespoons fresh basil or parsley leaves

1 tablespoon balsamic vinegar

1 tablespoon olive oil

$\frac{1}{4}$ teaspoon salt

$\frac{1}{2}$ teaspoon hot red pepper sauce, or to taste

1. Cook edamame according to package directions. Drain well and set aside, reserving 1 rounded tablespoon for garnish.

2. In a blender (see food processor variation below), combine tomato juice, fresh tomato, and ice. Blend until smooth, about 1 minute. Add cucumber, bell pepper, scallions, basil, vinegar, oil, salt, and pepper sauce. Blend just until vegetables are coarsely chopped.

3. Add edamame and blend again until coarsely chopped. Ladle into bowls, top with reserved edamame, and serve.

Make-Ahead Tip: Gazpacho can be made up to eight hours ahead and refrigerated.

Food Processor Variation: Prepare edamame as instructed in step 1. Place tomato juice in a large bowl. In a food processor, puree fresh tomatoes with 3 crushed ice cubes until smooth. Add to tomato juice in bowl. In a food processor, coarsely chop together cucumber, bell pepper, scallions, basil, and edamame. Add to tomato juice in bowl along with remaining ingredients, and stir to combine.

Chilled Cantaloupe Soup with Lime

A mug of this antioxidant-rich soup during hot weather is quite refreshing. Opening a whole bottle of wine for such a small amount may seem extravagant—and it can be eliminated—but it does make a difference in the flavor. And you can always share the rest of the bottle with others. The range of measurements given for some of the ingredients allows you to adjust the soup to suit your own taste. Try substituting other melons, such as honeydew or Persian. The coconut milk carries with it a little saturated fat, but the flavor is well worth it.

Serving Suggestions: Serve as a first course for a summer meal, then follow with Three Bean Salad with Edamame (page 129).

MAKES 4 SERVINGS
Prep: 10 minutes / Refrigerate: 2 hours

2 ripe cantaloupes

3 tablespoons white wine (optional)

2 to 3 tablespoons freshly squeezed lime juice

2 tablespoons orange juice

3 to 4 tablespoons canned regular or "lite" coconut milk

$\frac{1}{4}$ teaspoon salt

1. Cut cantaloupes in half. Scoop out and discard seeds, then scoop flesh into a food processor. Puree until very smooth. Transfer to a bowl and stir in remaining ingredients.
2. Refrigerate, tightly covered, until well chilled, about 2 hours.

Make-Ahead Tip: Soup can be refrigerated for up to a day.

Chilled Avocado Soup with Chiles and Lime

Recent studies about avocado have reported that it contains some compounds that may have prostate cancer–fighting properties. This soup is best served the same day made, since the avocado will begin to discolor slightly due to oxidation, even though the lime juice acts to retard the process.

Serving Suggestions: Accompany with an orange and red onion salad sprinkled with toasted sliced almonds and drizzled with a rice vinegar vinaigrette. Use the lesser amount of soy milk in the soup, and it will double as a dressing for fruit salads.

MAKES 4 SERVINGS
Prep: 15 minutes / Refrigerate: 1 hour

3 ripe avocados
$\frac{1}{2}$ cup vegetable broth, homemade (page 101) or store-bought
1–1$\frac{1}{2}$ cups unsweetened soy milk
1 can (4 ounces) chopped chiles
3 tablespoons freshly squeezed lime juice
$\frac{3}{4}$ teaspoon salt

1. Halve and pit avocados. Scoop out flesh into a food processor. Add broth and process until smooth. Add 1 cup soy milk, chiles, lime juice, and salt. Whirl again until smooth. For a thinner soup, while the motor is running, slowly pour the remaining soy milk through feed tube until it reaches the desired consistency.
2. Refrigerate until chilled, about 1 hour. Taste and adjust seasoning, adding more lime juice or salt if needed. Serve as soon as possible.

Make-Ahead Tip: The soup can be made earlier in the day and refrigerated. At the most, it can be refrigerated up to a day.

CHAPTER V

SALADS

VEGETABLES AND FRUIT

BROCCOLI AND ORANGE SALAD WITH WATER CHESTNUTS

TROPICAL FRUIT SALAD WITH AVOCADO

SPICY CABBAGE SALAD WITH CIDER VINEGAR

GREEK SALAD WITH MARINATED TOFU

ORZO SALAD WITH CARROT AND BROCCOLI

SWEET POTATO AND APPLE SALAD WITH ORANGE AND RED-WINE VINEGAR DRESSING

GERMAN POTATO SALAD WITH EDAMAME

ORANGE AND WATERCRESS SALAD WITH GINGER-MUSTARD DRESSING

WARM SCALLOP AND VEGETABLE SALAD WITH EDAMAME

LEGUMES AND GRAINS

SOYBEAN SALAD WITH SWEET PICKLE

THREE-BEAN SALAD WITH EDAMAME

RED LENTIL, SWEET POTATO, AND CHICKPEA SALAD

LENTIL AND BULGHUR SALAD WITH CHERRY TOMATOES AND MARINATED TOFU

RED RICE SALAD WITH LIME-MUSTARD DRESSING

DRESSINGS

CHILE-CITRUS DRESSING

ORANGE AND RED-WINE VINEGAR DRESSING

CREAMY HONEY-MUSTARD DRESSING

HONEY-CILANTRO VINAIGRETTE

RUSSIAN DRESSING WITH CHILI SAUCE

THOUSAND ISLAND DRESSING

TOMATO-BASIL DRESSING

GINGER-MUSTARD DRESSING

BALSAMIC VINAIGRETTE

ANTIOXIDANT HEAVEN (AS WELL AS FIBER)! Salads present a wealth of possibilities for combining ingredients beyond the usual lettuce. There are vegetables, fruits, legumes, grains, fish, and all kinds of newly available greens. Supermarket produce departments are now stocked with a large selection of prewashed, prebagged greens and salad mixes, some even organic, so the excuse "it takes too long to wash the greens" no longer works. If available, organic is best—less chance of pesticides and genetically modified foods. Leftovers are often a good place to start when creating salads. If you're steaming or roasting vegetables—broccoli, cauliflower, green beans, asparagus, carrots, beets, or bell peppers—or cooking rice or barley or couscous or other grains or legumes, always plan on making a little extra for salad-making on another day.

Adding grated soy cheese (or cubes or matchsticks) with its protein is an easy way to pump up a salad to entree status. Cow or goat milk cheese should probably be avoided since there is some evidence that excessive calcium in the diet may not be prostate friendly. The variety of soy cheeses increases practically daily and includes blocks, slices, and already-grated.

Shelled edamame, or green soybeans—an excellent source of soy protein and isoflavones—fresh or thawed frozen, are an easy addition to any salad, whether it's just a simple collection of greens or a combination of vegetables, grains, and legumes.

The calorie culprit in salads is often the dressing, since oil is fat. The good news is that the fat is monounsaturated and polyunsaturated and is thought to lower blood cholesterol. And remember that any heart-healthy food will in most cases be prostate-healthy too. If the dressings you make have a lot of flavor—such as Balsamic Vinaigrette (page 141), Orange and Red-Wine Vinegar Dressing (page 134), and Ginger-Mustard Dressing (page 140)—a little will go a long way. For creamy dressings, such as Creamy Honey-Mustard Dressing (page 135), silken tofu replaces oil, and the tofu can be pureed with a variety of ingredients for flavoring. The same holds true for eggless soy-based mayonnaise. And in both cases, the added bonus is the isoflavones from the soy, which are thought by some to have prostate cancer-fighting properties.

Broccoli and Orange Salad with Water Chestnuts

There are lots of antioxidants as well as 3 grams of fiber in this salad. And, if you leave some of the white pith and peel on the orange segments, you'll include citrus pectin (page 29), thought by some to have prostate cancer-fighting properties.

Serving Suggestions: Pair this with Pumpkin Polenta with Wild Mushroom Ragout (page 150), or a sandwich-soup combo.

MAKES 4 SERVINGS

Prep: 15 minutes / Cook: 3 minutes

> 1 small head broccoli, stalks removed and reserved for other use, head separated into small florets
> 1 navel orange, peeled, halved lengthwise, and cut crosswise into $\frac{1}{4}$-inch-thick slices
> Honey-Cilantro Vinaigrette (page 136)
> $\frac{1}{2}$ small red onion, cut crosswise into thin slices and separated
> 2 whole canned water chestnuts, thinly sliced
> $\frac{1}{4}$ teaspoon black pepper

1. In a large pot of lightly salted boiling water, cook broccoli florets until barely crisp-tender, 2 to 3 minutes Drain in colander. Rinse under cold running water to stop cooking.

2. In a large bowl, combine broccoli and orange with vinaigrette and toss to coat ingredients. Arrange on plates. Top with onion and water chestnuts. Sprinkle with pepper.

Make-Ahead Tip: All the ingredients, including vinaigrette, can be prepared several hours ahead and refrigerated separately. To serve, let come to room temperature and assemble.

Tropical Fruit Salad with Avocado

Molly McQuillan, one of my youngest taste-testers, dubbed this dish "waterfall salad" because you pour all the dressing over the entire salad just before serving. Even though it is relatively high in fat because of the avocado, researchers recently have suggested that avocado has cancer-fighting properties. There are 8 grams of fiber in this salad.

Serving Suggestions: To turn this into a main dish salad, add cubes of mozzarella-style or provolone-style soy cheese. You can also substitute diced apples, orange slices, halved cherry tomatoes, or cubes of honeydew melon for some of the fruits called for. Toss in a few chopped pickled jalapeños, for a little extra zip. This pairs well with Curried Brown Basmati Rice Pilaf with Vegetables (page 251).

MAKES 6 SERVINGS

Prep: 15 minutes

> 12 inner leaves Romaine lettuce, torn into bite-size pieces
>
> 2 firm ripe avocados, peeled, pitted, and cubed
>
> 2 celery stalks, thinly sliced
>
> 2 cups fresh pineapple cubes
>
> 2 cups watermelon cubes
>
> 1 large, firm ripe banana, peeled and cut into coins and tossed with lemon juice
>
> 1 pint strawberries, hulled and thickly sliced
>
> Chile-Citrus Dressing (page 133)

1. In a large shallow bowl or deep dish, arrange lettuce leaves.

2. In another large bowl, combine avocados, celery, pineapple, watermelon, banana, and strawberries. Spoon over lettuce. Pour dressing over top just before serving.

Make-Ahead Tip: Dressing can be made up to two days ahead and refrigerated.

Spicy Cabbage Salad with Cider Vinegar

Inspired by Asian pickled vegetables, this no-fat salad could be considered a version of sweet-and-sour coleslaw. Cabbage, a cruciferous vegetable, is touted by many as one of the major "super foods" with lots of anticancer properties. Because this salad is strongly flavored, a little may be sufficient for some people. For a more subtle flavor, substitute rice vinegar for the cider vinegar and omit the chile paste. For a really crunchy salad, cook the cabbage very, very briefly. The acid from the vinegar will soften the cabbage as it sits for a day or two.

Serving Suggestions: Serve as a side salad with a strong-flavored fish such as bluefish or salmon. It's also good as a sandwich topper wherever you might use coleslaw—try it with a Chickpea Burger with Almonds and Ginger (page 88) or Red Bean and Brazil Nut Burger with Rosemary (page 90).

MAKES 8 SERVINGS
Prep: 10 minutes / Cook: 2–8 minutes

> 1 small green cabbage (about 2 pounds), halved, cored, and thinly sliced or cut into small dice
> 2 to 3 teaspoons Asian chile paste or bottled red or green Thai curry paste
> $\frac{1}{2}$ cup cider vinegar
> 1 teaspoon salt
> $\frac{1}{8}$ teaspoon black pepper

1. Bring a large pot of water to a boil. Add cabbage and cook until desired degree of crisp-tenderness, 2 to 8 minutes. Drain well in colander.

2. In the bottom of a large bowl, stir together chile paste and 2 tablespoons of the vinegar until well blended. Stir in the remaining vinegar and the salt and pepper. Add cabbage and toss to thoroughly combine.

Make-Ahead Tip: Cabbage can be refrigerated for up to four days.

Greek Salad with Marinated Tofu

Feta cheese is very popular in Greek cuisine, but in this salad, crumbled marinated tofu replaces it, and you would never know! If you like, you can substitute an equal amount of feta-style soy cheese. Most of the fat here is monounsaturated from the olive oil used to marinate the tofu.

Serving Suggestions: Crispy bread sticks or slices of crusty bread would be a simple go-with.

MAKES 4 SERVINGS

Prep: 10 minutes / Marinate: 30 minutes:

> Greek-Style Marinated Tofu (page 66)
> 2 cups finely chopped Romaine lettuce
> 1 cucumber, peeled, halved lengthwise, seeded, and sliced crosswise
> 1 large ripe tomato, cored, halved, seeded, and chopped
> 1 small red onion, halved and thinly sliced crosswise
> $\frac{1}{2}$ red or green bell pepper, cored, seeded, and chopped
> 12 pitted black Greek olives, halved

In a large bowl, combine all the ingredients and toss gently. Serve at once.

Orzo Salad with Carrot and Broccoli

Orzo is a rice-shaped pasta that makes a delicious starting point for all kinds of salads. For a Mediterranean flair, sprinkle with feta-style soy cheese or Greek-Style Marinated Tofu (page 66). Fresh fennel is crunchy like celery with the flavor of licorice and in most places it's available all year round.

Serving Suggestions: Serve for lunch or a light supper with a crusty whole-wheat baguette and sliced tomatoes. It's also a nice complement to a mild-flavored fish dish such as Flounder with Fennel and Lemon (page 197).

MAKES 4 SERVINGS
Prep: 15 minutes / Cook: 10 minutes

$1\frac{1}{4}$ cups orzo

About 2 cups vegetable broth, homemade (page 101) or store-bought

2 cups broccoli florets (1 small head)

2 carrots, trimmed, peeled, and diced

$\frac{1}{2}$ fennel bulb, cored and diced

4 scallions, trimmed and chopped

2 tablespoons olive oil

3 tablespoons balsamic vinegar or red-wine vinegar

1 tablespoon Dijon mustard

2 teaspoons grated orange zest

$\frac{1}{2}$ teaspoon salt

$\frac{1}{4}$ teaspoon black pepper

$\frac{1}{4}$ cup fresh basil leaves, cut into thin strips (optional)

1. Cook orzo according to the package directions, replacing one quarter of the cooking water with vegetable broth. Drain in a colander and rinse under cold water to stop cooking. Shake colander well to remove excess water and transfer orzo to a large bowl.

2. Meanwhile, in a large saucepan fitted with a steamer basket, bring 1 inch water to a boil. Add broccoli, cover, and cook until crisp-tender, about 3 minutes. Drain and rinse under cold water to stop cooking. Shake to remove excess water and add to orzo along with carrots, fennel, and scallions.

3. In a small bowl, whisk together oil, vinegar, mustard, zest, salt, and pepper. Stir in basil if using. Pour dressing over orzo mixture. Gently stir to coat orzo and vegetables. Serve at room temperature or chilled.

Make-Ahead Tip: Salad can be prepared up to two days ahead and refrigerated. If the salad seems a little dry, make another batch of the vinegar dressing mixture and slowly drizzle it over the salad as needed.

Sweet Potato and Apple Salad with Orange and Red-Wine Vinegar Dressing

Using sweet potatoes, rich in antioxidants, is a nutritionally smart alternative to the white potato in a traditional potato salad. The recipe also capitalizes on the antioxidants in watercress.

Serving Suggestions: Serve as a salad accompaniment to a bowl of Mexican Corn Stew with Red Beans and Chiles (page 104), Baked Tuna with Honey Glaze and Moroccan Spices (page 190), or your favorite sandwich.

MAKES 6 SERVINGS
Prep: 15 minutes / Cook: 15 minutes

> $1\frac{1}{2}$ pounds sweet potatoes, peeled and cut into cubes
>
> 1 Granny Smith apple, peeled, cored, and cut into cubes
>
> 3 scallions, trimmed and finely chopped
>
> Orange and Red-Wine Vinegar Dressing (page 134)
>
> 1 bunch watercress, tough stems removed
>
> 1 small Belgian endive, cored and separated into leaves

1. Bring a large pot of water to a boil. Add sweet potato cubes and cook until crisp-tender, 10 to 15 minutes. Shake the excess water from the colander.

2. In a large bowl, combine sweet potato, apple, and scallions. Add half of the dressing and toss to coat.

3. In a separate bowl, toss together watercress and remaining dressing.

4. To assemble salad, place watercress on serving platter or salad plates. Arrange sweet potato mixture on top along with endive leaves.

German Potato Salad with Edamame

The flavor of bacon is here as in the traditional version, but without the fat since you use soy bacon. Edamame adds a little color as well as protein—9 grams total in this salad.

Serving Suggestions: This salad would be the perfect match with any of the veggie burgers (pages 88–91), or serve it on its own, paired with a simple green salad and breadsticks.

MAKES 6 SERVINGS
Prep: 20 minutes / Cook: 15 minutes

$1\frac{1}{2}$ pounds Yukon gold potatoes, unpeeled and cut into $\frac{3}{4}$-inch chunks

$\frac{2}{3}$ cup frozen shelled and blanched edamame

$1\frac{1}{2}$ tablespoons olive oil

6 large shallots, thickly sliced crosswise, or 1 bunch scallions, trimmed and thinly sliced

4 strips soy bacon ($1\frac{1}{2}$ ounces), cut into $\frac{1}{2}$-inch squares (halve lengthwise, cut crosswise into $\frac{1}{2}$-inch pieces)

3 tablespoons cider vinegar

1 tablespoon honey

2 teaspoons coarse-grained Dijon mustard

$\frac{1}{4}$ teaspoon salt

$\frac{1}{8}$ teaspoon black pepper

1. Place potatoes in a pot with enough cold water to cover. Bring to a boil. Lower heat and simmer for 4 minutes. Add edamame and simmer until potatoes are tender when pierced with a knife, about 4 more minutes. Drain well in a colander, reserving about $\frac{1}{2}$ cup of the cooking liquid.

2. Meanwhile, in a large nonstick skillet, heat oil over medium heat. Add shallots and cook, stirring occasionally, until softened and golden brown, about 6 minutes. Add bacon and cook, stirring, for 1 minute more. Remove from heat.

3. Stir vinegar, honey, mustard, salt, and pepper into the skillet. Add $\frac{1}{4}$ cup of the potato water and stir to combine. Add the potato mixture and toss until well combined. If salad seems a little dry, add additional potato cooking liquid by the tablespoon. Serve warm.

Make-Ahead Tip: Potato salad can be refrigerated for up to three days. Serve chilled, at room temperature, or gently rewarm in a large skillet or microwave on medium power.

Orange and Watercress Salad with Ginger-Mustard Dressing

The hallmark of this salad is its tingly sharp flavors, as well as its wealth of antioxidants.

Serving Suggestions: Pair it with strongly flavored fish entrees such as Broiled Salmon with Cumin and Lemon (page 192) or Soy-Glazed Halibut with Shiitake Mushrooms (page 207), or with vegetarian entrees such as Fennel and Chickpea Stew with Apricots and Raisins (page 156) or Red Lentil and Sweet Potato Stew with Indian Spices (page 168).

MAKES 4 SERVINGS
Prep: 15 minutes

   1 bunch watercress, tough stems removed

   2 bunches arugula, trimmed

   1 small cucumber, halved lengthwise, seeded, and cut crosswise into thin slices

   1 navel orange, peeled, halved lengthwise, and thinly sliced crosswise

   4 slices red onion, separated into rings

   $\frac{1}{4}$ cup Ginger-Mustard Dressing (page 140)

Arrange the watercress, arugula, cucumber, orange, and onion on salad plates. Drizzle 1 tablespoon of dressing over each salad.

Make-Ahead Tip: The watercress and arugula can be washed and trimmed a day ahead and refrigerated separately in plastic bags.

Warm Scallop and Vegetable Salad with Edamame

The edamame adds a touch of green as well protective isoflavones. Once all the vegetables are prepped, the cooking and assembly take very little time.

Serving Suggestions: To finish the picture, serve a basket of Homemade Crostini (page 56) with Roasted Garlic (page 261), and a glass of a dry white wine, such as chenin blanc, pinot gris, or chardonnay.

MAKES 4 MAIN COURSE OR 8 APPETIZER SERVINGS
Prep: 20 minutes / Cook: 8 minutes

> 6 cups mixed salad greens (your own mix or store-bought prepackaged)
>
> 2 cups (about 6 ounces) thinly sliced fennel
>
> 1 pound sea scallops, side muscle removed and scallops blotted dry with paper towels
>
> $1\frac{1}{2}$ teaspoons grated lemon zest
>
> $\frac{1}{4}$ teaspoon salt
>
> $\frac{1}{4}$ teaspoon black pepper
>
> 2 tablespoons olive oil
>
> $\frac{1}{3}$ cup vegetable broth, homemade (page 101) or store-bought
>
> $\frac{3}{4}$ cup frozen shelled and blanched edamame, thawed
>
> 1 small red bell pepper, cored, seeded, and cut into thin, 2-inch-long slivers
>
> 2 scallions, trimmed and cut into thin, 2-inch-long slivers
>
> 1 tablespoon sherry vinegar
>
> $\frac{1}{2}$ teaspoon honey

1. Divide salad greens and fennel among four salad plates. In a medium-size bowl, toss together scallops, 1 teaspoon of the lemon zest, and $\frac{1}{8}$ teaspoon each of salt and pepper.
2. In a large nonstick skillet, heat 1 tablespoon of the olive oil over medium-high heat. Add scallops and cook, turning over when browned, just until they turn opaque in the center, 2 to 3 minutes—do not overcook. Transfer scallops to a plate and cover to keep warm.

3. Add broth, edamame, and bell pepper to the skillet and bring to a simmer. Cover and cook until vegetables are crisp-tender, about 4 minutes. Stir in scallions and cook for 1 minute. Remove the skillet from the heat and stir in vinegar, honey, the remaining 1 tablespoon oil, $\frac{1}{2}$ teaspoon lemon zest, and $\frac{1}{8}$ teaspoon each salt and pepper. Stir in any juices from scallops.

4. Divide scallops over the greens on the salad plates and top with warm vegetables and dressing. Serve immediately.

Make-Ahead Tip: The vegetables can be prepped earlier in the day, bagged, and refrigerated.

Soybean Salad with Sweet Pickle

The soybeans in this easy-to-fix salad provide protein—7 grams per serving—as well as isoflavones.

Serving Suggestions: In five minutes you can prepare this salad to serve with veggie burgers (pages 88–91) or on its own as a snack. For a light lunch, spoon into hollowed-out tomatoes or spears of Belgian endive, or wrap it in Romaine lettuce leaves to make little packets.

MAKES 4 SERVINGS

Prep: 5 minutes

   1 can (15 ounces) yellow soybeans, drained and rinsed
   $\frac{1}{4}$ cup finely chopped scallions (about 6 scallions)
   2 tablespoons chopped sweet pickle or pickle relish
   $\frac{1}{4}$ teaspoon salt
   $\frac{1}{4}$ teaspoon black pepper
   $\frac{1}{4}$ cup eggless soy-based mayonnaise

In a medium-size bowl, combine all the ingredients. Refrigerate until chilled.

Make-Ahead Tip: Salad can be refrigerated for up to two days.

Three-Bean Salad with Edamame

An American classic, sweetened with a little honey and updated with edamame for 4 grams of protein per serving at only 110 calories. This is a great summer salad for a crowd, or halve the amounts for a modest-size crew.

Serving Suggestions: Serve with a Salmon Salad Sandwich with Red Bell Pepper (page 81) or a Tuna Fish Salad Sandwich with Scallions and Pickled Ginger (page 82). Or, put together a snack plate that includes Homemade Crostini (page 56), or Homemade Pita Chips (page 53) with Tuna and White Bean Spread with Lemon and Rosemary (page 46).

MAKES 8 SERVINGS
Prep: 15 minutes / Cook: 7 minutes / Refrigerate: 3 hours

> $\frac{1}{2}$ pound green beans, trimmed and cut into 1-inch pieces
>
> 1 cup frozen shelled and blanched edamame
>
> $\frac{1}{2}$ small red onion, chopped
>
> $\frac{1}{3}$ cup red wine vinegar or cider vinegar
>
> 2 tablespoons olive oil
>
> 1 tablespoon honey
>
> 2 teaspoons Dijon mustard
>
> $\frac{1}{2}$ teaspoon salt
>
> 1 can (15 ounces) chickpeas, rinsed and drained
>
> $\frac{1}{2}$ red bell pepper, cored, seeded, and chopped

1. Bring a large saucepan filled with water to a boil. Add green beans and cook until almost tender, about 5 minutes. Add edamame and cook until beans and edamame are tender, about 2 minutes more.

2. Meanwhile, place onion in a colander in the sink. Drain beans and boiling water over onion and rinse with cold running water. Drain well.

3. In a large bowl, whisk together vinegar, oil, honey, mustard, and salt. Add chickpeas, bell pepper, and green bean mixture and toss to combine. Spoon into a plastic food storage bag, push out all the air, and seal. Refrigerate for at least 3 hours or up to 24 hours before serving.

Make-Ahead Tip: Salad can be made up to a day ahead—longer than that and the flavor loses its brightness.

Red Lentil, Sweet Potato, and Chickpea Salad

This creamy main-dish salad is a primer on how to make exciting food with big taste to make up for the absence of fat. The combination of lemon, fresh ginger, Dijon mustard, chutney, and apple makes for a lively tart-sweet flavor. If you've never tried soy yogurt, this is a good time to sneak it in under the radar, as it were. There is enough nonanimal protein here from the red lentils and chickpeas (12 grams per serving) to make the salad a main course, and the lentils contribute to the 10 grams of fiber. Plus, there are only 2 grams of fat and lots of antioxidants from the sweet potato.

Serving Suggestions: For crunch, accompany with low-fat thin wheat crackers or crispy flat bread, homemade (page 54) or store-bought.

MAKES 4 SERVINGS

Prep: 15 minutes / Cook: 10 minutes

  2 sweet potatoes, peeled and cut into $\frac{1}{2}$-inch chunks

  $\frac{1}{2}$ cup dried red lentils, picked over and rinsed

  $\frac{3}{4}$ cup plain soy yogurt

  2 tablespoons bottled mango chutney, big pieces chopped

  1 tablespoon freshly squeezed lemon juice

  2 teaspoons peeled, finely chopped fresh ginger

  2 teaspoons Dijon mustard

  $\frac{1}{2}$ teaspoon salt

  $\frac{1}{4}$ teaspoon black pepper

  4 scallions, trimmed and thinly sliced

  1 Granny Smith apple, with or without skin, cored, and cut into $\frac{1}{2}$-inch chunks

  1 can (15 ounces) chickpeas, drained and rinsed

1. Bring a large pot of water to a boil. Add sweet potatoes and cook for 5 minutes. Add lentils and boil until potatoes and lentils are tender, about another 5 minutes. Drain very well.

2. In a large bowl, whisk together soy yogurt, chutney, lemon juice, ginger, mustard, salt, and pepper. Fold in scallions, apple, chickpeas, and potato-lentil mixture. Serve at room temperature.

Make-Ahead Tip: Salad can be refrigerated for up to three days. If it becomes a little too dry while sitting in the refrigerator, remoisten with a little soy yogurt.

Lentil and Bulghur Salad with Cherry Tomatoes and Marinated Tofu

The combination of the lentils with the bulghur and tofu makes for a very "meaty" salad, and a good source of nonanimal-based protein (about 12 grams per serving).

Serving Suggestions: Keep it simple—slices of crusty whole-grain bread, drizzled with a little extra-virgin olive oil or spread with Roasted Garlic (page 261).

MAKES 4 SERVINGS
Prep: 35 minutes / Cook: 15 minutes

$^3/_4$ cup fine-grain bulghur wheat

$^1/_2$ teaspoon salt

$^1/_4$ teaspoon black pepper

$^3/_4$ cup dried brown lentils, picked over and rinsed

$^1/_4$ cup freshly squeezed lemon juice

2 tablespoons olive oil

$^1/_2$ teaspoon dried rosemary

2 cups (1 pint) cherry tomatoes, each halved

4 scallions, trimmed and thinly sliced

1 cup Greek-Style Marinated Tofu (page 66) or crumbled feta-style soy cheese

1 cup pitted black olives (optional)

1. In a small saucepan, bring 1 cup water to a boil. Stir in bulghur, salt, and pepper. Cover pan, remove from heat, and let stand until water is absorbed, about 30 minutes.

2. Meanwhile, in a medium-size saucepan, cover lentils with water by 1 inch. Bring to a boil. Reduce heat and simmer, covered, until lentils are tender but firm, about 15 minutes. Drain well.

3. In a large bowl, stir together lemon juice, olive oil, and rosemary.

4. Spoon bulghur into lemon juice mixture. Gently fold in lentils, tomatoes, and scallions until evenly coated. Sprinkle top with marinated tofu, and olives if using, and serve.

Make-Ahead Tip: The lentil mixture can be refrigerated for up to two days. Top salad with tofu and olives just before serving.

Red Rice Salad with Lime-Mustard Dressing

Supermarket shelves are full of different kinds of rice these days, so there is no reason to be stuck on refined white rice, which lacks some nutrients since the hull and germ have been removed. The Butan red rice in this recipe has a sweet, nutty flavor, with a slightly chewy texture.

Serving Suggestions: The salad is delicious with pan-seared fish fillets or on its own as a snack, scooped up with tortilla chips and crispy wheat thins. Or spoon it into hollowed-out cherry tomatoes.

MAKES 4 SERVINGS
Prep: 10 minutes / Cook: 20 minutes

1 bay leaf

1 cup butan red rice

$\frac{1}{4}$ cup freshly squeezed lime juice (2–4 limes)

2 teaspoons Dijon mustard

1 tablespoon olive oil

$\frac{1}{2}$ teaspoon salt, or to taste

$\frac{1}{4}$ teaspoon black pepper, or to taste

$\frac{1}{2}$ small red bell pepper, cored, seeded, and finely chopped

3 scallions, trimmed and thinly sliced

1 plum tomato, canned or fresh, cut into small dice

1. In a small saucepan, bring $1\frac{1}{2}$ cups of water and bay leaf to a boil. Stir in rice. Reduce heat to low and simmer, covered, until rice is tender and water is absorbed, 20 minutes.

2. Meanwhile, in a medium-size bowl, whisk together lime juice, mustard, oil, salt, and pepper. Remove about half of the dressing to a small bowl and set aside.

3. When rice is done, scrape into the medium-size bowl with dressing and remove the bay leaf. Gently stir with rubber spatula to coat rice. Let cool at room temperature.

4. Add bell pepper, scallions, and tomato and fold together gently. Taste the salad, and if it's too dry, add a little more dressing. Add more salt and pepper, if needed.

Make-Ahead Tip: Salad can be refrigerated for up to three days. Add more dressing if too dry.

Chile-Citrus Dressing

Add as much chili powder as you like to this dressing, with its combination of three citrus juices.

Serving Suggestions: The sharp citrus flavors blend well in fruit salads or with assertive greens such as chicory and watercress.

MAKES ABOUT $\frac{1}{3}$ CUP
Prep: 5 minutes

$\frac{1}{4}$ cup olive oil

2 tablespoons orange juice

1 tablespoon freshly squeezed lemon juice

1 tablespoon pineapple juice

$\frac{1}{2}$ teaspoon Dijon mustard

$\frac{1}{2}$ teaspoon organic sugar (evaporated cane juice)

$\frac{1}{4}$ teaspoon salt

Pinch chili powder, or more to taste

In a small bowl, whisk together all the ingredients, or shake together in a glass jar with a screw-top lid.

Make-Ahead Tip: Dressing can be refrigerated for up to three days.

Orange and Red-Wine Vinegar Dressing

A sharp-tasting dressing that will perk up any salad.

Serving Suggestions: Toss with a fruit salad; mix with assertive greens, such as escarole, arugula, or mustard greens; or drizzle over cooked vegetables, such as broccoli, Brussels sprouts, or green beans.

MAKES ABOUT $\frac{1}{3}$ CUP
Prep: 5 minutes

  3 tablespoons red-wine vinegar
  2 teaspoons grated orange zest
  3 tablespoons freshly squeezed orange juice
  Pinch salt
  2 tablespoons olive oil

In a small bowl, whisk together all the ingredients, or shake together in a glass jar with a screw-top lid.

Make-Ahead Tip: Dressing can be refrigerated for up to three days.

Creamy Honey-Mustard Dressing

Silken tofu adds the creamy texture, with only 1 gram of fat per tablespoon and no saturated fat. The dressing is sweetened with a combination of honey and maple syrup.

Serving Suggestions: Spoon over fruit salads and green salads, burgers on their own without the bun (pages 88-91), and cooked vegetables such as sliced carrots.

MAKES ABOUT 1 CUP
Prep: 5 minutes / Refrigerate: 2 hours

6 ounces silken tofu, drained and blotted dry with paper towels

2–3 tablespoons Dijon mustard

2 tablespoons honey

2 tablespoons maple syrup

2 teaspoons freshly squeezed lemon juice

$\frac{1}{4}$ teaspoon salt

1. In a small food processor or blender, puree tofu. Add mustard, honey, maple syrup, lemon juice, and salt. Process to a smooth puree, scraping down the sides of the work bowl as needed.

2. Transfer to a glass jar with a screw-top lid, or other container, and refrigerate for 2 hours to mellow mustard flavor and firm up texture.

Make-Ahead Tip: Dressing can be refrigerated for up to three days.

Honey-Cilantro Vinaigrette

The orange juice and honey sweetly counter the soy and vinegar.

Serving Suggestions: Drizzle over fruit salads with papaya or mango or melons, or vegetable salads, such as shredded carrots with chopped scallions and radishes, or broccoli and sliced water chestnuts. Very tasty mixed with assertive greens such as escarole, arugula, or watercress.

MAKES ⅓ CUP
Prep: 5 minutes

    2 tablespoons orange juice
    2 teaspoons honey
    2 teaspoons soy sauce
    1 teaspoon cider vinegar
    2 tablespoons olive oil
    1 tablespoon chopped fresh cilantro, or 1 teaspoon ground cumin

In a small bowl, whisk together all the ingredients, or shake together in a glass jar with a screw-top lid.

Make-Ahead Tip: Dressing, without the fresh cilantro, can be refrigerated for up to three days. Add cilantro just before serving.

Russian Dressing with Chili Sauce

This favorite from the 1950s is nutritionally updated, with eggless soy-based mayonnaise and soy yogurt replacing the traditional fat-laden ingredients.

Serving Suggestions: Delicious tossed with vegetable salads made with broccoli, Brussels sprouts, or cauliflower, spooned over sliced tomatoes, or used as a sandwich spread.

MAKES ABOUT ¾ CUP
Prep: 5 minutes

   ⅓ cup eggless soy-based mayonnaise
   ⅓ cup plain soy yogurt
   4 teaspoons bottled chili sauce
   2 tablespoons finely chopped scallions
   2 teaspoons Dijon mustard
   ¼ teaspoon salt
   ⅛ teaspoon black pepper

In a blender or small food processor, combine all ingredients and blend until smooth, scraping down the sides of the bowl as needed.

Make-Ahead Tip: Dressing can be refrigerated for up to three days.

Thousand Island Dressing

An American favorite, good practically anywhere, anytime, but especially yummy over a wedge of iceberg lettuce, or better yet, dark leafy greens. This soy version has about half as much fat as the store-bought variety, and with the added bonus of isoflavones from the soy.

Serving Suggestions: Spoon over vegetable salads or just plain blanched vegetables and use as a sandwich flavor-enchancer, as in a Reuben Sandwich with Sauerkraut and Thousand Island Dressing (page 76).

MAKES ABOUT 1 CUP
Prep: 5 minutes

$\frac{1}{2}$ cup eggless soy-based mayonnaise
$\frac{1}{4}$ cup soy yogurt
$\frac{1}{4}$ cup ketchup
2 tablespoons sweet pickle relish
$\frac{1}{8}$ teaspoon salt

In a small bowl, stir together all the ingredients.

Make-Ahead Tip: Dressing can be refrigerated for up to three days.

Tomato-Basil Dressing

Save this one for the summer, when basil is at its best. Without the addition of the olive oil, this dressing has a very bright taste. The oil thickens it and quiets the flavor.

Serving Suggestions: Drizzle over a simple green salad with the ripest tomatoes. Or toss the dressing, without the oil, with hot whole-wheat penne or rigatoni for a quick pasta dish.

MAKES ABOUT ¾ CUP
Prep: 5 minutes

> 6 sun-dried tomato halves, packed in oil
> 1 cup coarsely chopped tomato, fresh or canned
> ¼ cup coarsely chopped fresh basil
> 2 tablespoons balsamic vinegar
> ¼ teaspoon salt
> ⅛ teaspoon black pepper
> 2 tablespoons olive oil (optional)

In a blender or food processor, puree together sun-dried tomatoes, chopped tomato, basil, vinegar, salt, and pepper. If using oil, slowly add it with the machine running.

Make-Ahead Tip: Dressing can be refrigerated for up three days.

Ginger-Mustard Dressing

All the flavors in this dressing are evenly balanced. Rice vinegar has a more subtle flavor than other vinegar choices.

Serving Suggestions: Spoon over vegetable or fruit salads or a selection of assertive greens.

MAKES ABOUT $\frac{1}{4}$ CUP
Prep: 5 minutes

2 tablespoons rice vinegar

2 tablespoons freshly squeezed lemon juice

2 teaspoons Dijon mustard

1 teaspoon ground ginger

Pinch salt

Pinch black pepper

2 tablespoons light olive oil

In a small bowl, whisk together all the ingredients, or shake together in a glass jar with a screw-top lid.

Make-Ahead Tip: Dressing can be refrigerated for up to five days.

Balsamic Vinaigrette

This is a strongly flavored dressing, so a little goes along way. The Dijon mustard harmonizes with the tart-sweet balsamic vinegar. If the dressing is too tart for your taste, add a little more oil to soften the flavor, but remember, you're adding calories if you do (1 tablespoon oil contains 120 calories). However, on the good side, you're upping the amount of monounsaturated and polyunsaturated fat. You can easily double the recipe; keep the dressing on hand in the refrigerator for everyday use.

Serving Suggestions: Toss with greens, drizzle over sliced tomatoes, accent vegetable salads such as broccoli, cauliflower, carrot, and green bean, or even spoon a little over broiled fish.

MAKES ABOUT 6 TABLESPOONS
Prep: 5 minutes

$\frac{1}{4}$ cup balsamic vinegar
3 tablespoons olive oil
1 tablespoon Dijon mustard

In a small bowl, whisk together all the ingredients, or shake together in a glass jar with a screw-top lid.

Make-Ahead Tip: Dressing can be refrigerated for up to five days.

CHAPTER VI

VEGETARIAN MAIN DISHES

NONE OF THE RECIPES IN THIS COOKBOOK use beef, pork, or poultry, and that's part of my low-fat eating plan. In the midst of the growing discussion about the link between diet and prostate cancer, there is general agreement that low-fat menu planning may help to prevent the onset and retard the spread of the disease. And perhaps just as important, a reduced-fat diet is acknowledged as an important way to help prevent cardiovascular disease and diabetes.

Animal products, including dairy and eggs, contain arachidonic acid, a particular fatty acid that has been linked to the growth of prostate cancer cells. And even though only a small amount of this fat is found in poultry, I've decided not to include poultry recipes. I, in fact, do eat chicken from time to time, but I always steer toward skinless breasts. A recent lunch special on a budget airline was a very satisfying Asian chicken salad: marinated boneless, skinless chicken breasts, over a black rice salad with cranberries, and shredded red and green cabbage on the side—who says it's not possible to eat wisely when away from home?

In this chapter I rely on grains, legumes, and soy for sources of protein—and with these choices there is the added benefit of lots of soluble fiber. The Black Bean and Tortilla Casserole with Salsa (page 154) is one of my favorites—it tastes as though it's full of meat. A close second is the Nutty Lentil Loaf with Veggies and Mozzarella Cheese (page 158). And then there is Pumpkin Polenta with Wild Mushroom Ragout (page 150), Mac and Three Cheeses with Scallion and Tomato (page 180), Shepherd's Pie with Sweet Potato Topping (page 182), and an amazing Three-Mushroom Stroganoff with Thyme (page 179) made creamy with silken tofu.

Many of these dishes can be made when you have the time and then refrigerated for up to three days, and in some cases even frozen so when there is no time to cook, dinner just needs to be reheated.

Baked Rice and Jack Cheese Casserole with Chiles and Corn

This homey Tex-Mex style casserole is a good introduction to a variety of soy-based products: soy yogurt, soy milk, and soy cheese.

Serving Suggestions: An avocado and orange salad is a good match.

MAKES 6 SERVINGS

Prep: 15 minutes / Cook: 1 hour, 15 minutes

> 3 cups vegetable broth, homemade (page 101) or store-bought
> 1¾ cups brown rice
> 1 tablespoon olive oil
> 1 cup chopped scallions (about 1 bunch)
> ½ cup plain soy yogurt
> ½ cup unsweetened soy milk
> ½ teaspoon salt
> 2 cups (about 8 ounces) shredded Monterey Jack–style or pepper Jack–style soy cheese
> 1 cup bottled salsa
> 2 cups frozen corn kernels, thawed
> 1 can (4.5 ounces) diced chiles, or 1 canned chipotle in adobo, seeded and chopped
> ¼ cup chopped fresh cilantro (optional)
> Nonstick olive oil cooking spray
> 1 tomato, cored and sliced

1. In a medium-size saucepan, bring broth to a boil. Stir in rice, lower heat, cover, and simmer until tender, 40 to 45 minutes. Remove from heat and let stand for 5 minutes.

2. In a small skillet, heat oil over medium heat. And scallions and cook, stirring occasionally, until tender, about 3 minutes.

3. In a large bowl, stir together yogurt, soy milk, and salt. Stir in scallions, cheese, salsa, corn, chiles, rice, and cilantro, if using.

4. Heat oven to 350°F. Lightly coat 9 x 9 x 2-inch square baking dish with cooking spray. Scrape rice mixture into prepared dish and pat down. Arrange tomato slices on top.

5. Bake until golden brown on top and bubbly, 30 to 35 minutes. Let stand 10 minutes.

Make-Ahead Tip: Casserole can be assembled the day before and refrigerated. Leftovers can be reheated in a 350°F oven or microwave.

Barley Risotto with Asparagus and Wild Mushrooms

Barley replaces the Italian short-grained rice that is usually used for making risotto. You can substitute small broccoli florets or snow peas or cut-up green beans for the asparagus, adjusting the cooking time in step 3. This dish, like any risotto, requires some attended cooking on the stovetop, but the results are worth the effort—and there are 10 grams of fiber per serving. Leftover risotto can be shaped into small patties and pan-cooked in a skillet.

Serving Suggestions: To round out the menu, toss a prepackaged organic salad mix with Balsamic Vinaigrette (page 141) or your favorite low-fat dressing.

MAKES 4 SERVINGS

Prep: 15 minutes / Cook: 40 minutes

$3\frac{1}{2}$ cups vegetable broth, homemade (page 101) or store-bought

2 tablespoons olive oil

1 onion, finely chopped

8 ounces mushrooms, preferably a mixture of wild varieties, cleaned, tough stems removed, and mushrooms coarsely chopped

2 cloves garlic, finely chopped

1 cup pearl barley, rinsed

8 ounces fresh asparagus, preferably thin spears, trimmed, and cut into bite-size pieces, leaving tips whole

$\frac{3}{4}$ teaspoon dried sage

$\frac{1}{2}$ cup grated Parmesan-style soy cheese

1. In a saucepan, heat together the broth and 2 cups water to just below a simmer. Cover.

2. In a large, deep, nonstick skillet, heat oil over medium heat. Add onion and cook, stirring occasionally, until slightly softened, 3 minutes. Add mushrooms and garlic and cook, stirring occasionally, until mushrooms are softened, 5 minutes. Stir in barley and 2 cups hot broth mixture. Cover and simmer until most of the liquid is absorbed, 15 minutes.

3. Meanwhile, in the pot of hot broth mixture, blanch asparagus until crisp-tender, about 2 minutes. Using a slotted spoon, transfer asparagus to a plate.

4. Add more hot broth to barley mixture, $\frac{1}{2}$ cup at a time, stirring frequently. Let each batch of liquid be absorbed before adding more. When adding the last batch of liquid, stir in asparagus stem pieces, reserving the tips. When mixture is creamy and barley firm but tender, about 40 minutes total, remove saucepan from heat. Stir in sage and Parmesan. Serve risotto topped with asparagus tips.

Barley with Black Beans and Roasted Peppers

This robustly flavored grain and bean dish is really a salad that is tossed with a balsamic vinegar and oregano dressing. See the suggestions below for add-ins. The barley and black beans combine for complete protein, and for each serving, there are 9 grams of fiber, with 3 grams of monounsaturated and polyunsaturated fat, and no saturated fat. For an extra protein boost, you can add 12 ounces of firm tofu, cubed, in step 3 along with the black beans. Any leftovers keep very well.

Serving Suggestions: For a tart accompaniment, toss some sliced Granny Smith apples with a citrus vinaigrette and arrange on baby spinach leaves. If you would like another dish or two for this meal, try the Broccoli Rabe with Garlic and Parmesan Cheese (page 232) and Lima Beans with Sage (page 238).

MAKES 6 SERVINGS

Prep: 15 minutes / Cook: 40 minutes

Juice of half lemon (about 2 tablespoons)

2 tablespoons balsamic vinegar

1 tablespoon olive oil

1 tablespoon dried oregano

$\frac{3}{4}$ teaspoon salt

$\frac{1}{4}$ teaspoon black pepper

3 cups vegetable broth, homemade (page 101) or store-bought

1 cup pearl barley, rinsed

1 can (19 ounces) black beans, drained and rinsed

1 jar (12 ounces) roasted red bell peppers, drained and sliced

1 cup sliced scallions (about 1 bunch)

$\frac{1}{4}$ cup chopped flat-leaf parsley (optional)

1. In a large bowl, whisk together lemon juice, vinegar, olive oil, oregano, salt, and pepper. Set aside.

2. In a large saucepan, bring vegetable broth to a boil. Stir in barley. Cover, reduce heat to low, and simmer until broth is absorbed and barley is tender, about 30 minutes. Let stand, covered, for 10 minutes. Drain, if necessary.

3. Add barley to dressing in bowl. Fold in black beans, roasted peppers, scallions, and parsley if using. Serve warm or at room temperature.

Add-Ins: When you add the black beans in step 3, you can also add one or all of the following: 1 cup corn kernels, fresh or thawed frozen; 1 cup thawed frozen green peas; 1 cup chopped ripe tomato. For each add-in, you increase the yield by one serving.

Make-Ahead Tip: The dish can be refrigerated for up to two days. Taste and adjust seasonings before serving, adding more vinegar or lemon juice as needed. Gently rewarm or serve at room temperature.

Curried Bulghur with Tomatoes and Chickpeas

Bulghur is a nutritious substitution for white rice, and it actually cooks a bit faster. In this recipe, bottled chutney adds a touch of sweetness to the grain. It's worth mentioning that there are 12 grams of fiber per serving. Add 12 ounces of firm tofu, cubed, and you increase the amount of protein. The curried bulghur can also be served over whole-grain couscous or a whole-wheat shaped pasta such as rotelle or rigatoni.

Serving Suggestions: If there are any leftovers, combine the chickpea mixture and bulghur, chill, and serve as a salad with sandwiches or for snacking. Options for side dishes as part of the main meal include Broccoli Rabe with Garlic and Parmesan Cheese (page 232), or Sauteed Lima Beans and Spinach with Red Bell Pepper (page 239).

MAKES 6 SERVINGS
Prep: 10 minutes / Cook: 15 minutes

  $1\frac{1}{2}$ cups bulghur

  $\frac{1}{2}$ cup golden raisins

  1 cinnamon stick, broken

  2 cups vegetable broth, homemade (page 101) or store-bought, or water

  1 can (19 ounces) chickpeas, drained and rinsed

  3 fresh tomatoes, cored and diced, or 1 can (14.5 ounces) diced tomatoes

  1 carrot, trimmed, peeled, and cut into small dice

  2 teaspoons curry powder

  $\frac{1}{4}$ teaspoon salt

  $\frac{1}{4}$ cup bottled chutney, large pieces chopped

  1 tablespoon Dijon mustard

1. In a medium-size saucepan, combine bulghur, raisins, cinnamon stick, and broth. Cover and bring to a boil. Lower heat and gently simmer until water is absorbed, about 15 minutes.
2. Meanwhile, in a second saucepan, combine chickpeas, tomatoes, carrot, curry powder, and salt. Bring to a simmer and gently cook until carrot pieces are tender and mixture is heated through, 5 to 10 minutes. Keep warm.
3. When bulghur is ready, remove cinnamon stick. Stir in chutney and mustard.
4. To serve, spoon bulghur onto plates and top with chickpea mixture.

Make-Ahead Tip: Chickpea mixture and bulghur can be refrigerated separately for up to two days. Gently reheat each in a saucepan to serve, adding more broth if necessary.

Quinoa with Mushrooms and Red Bell Pepper

Quinoa is a protein-dense grain (for more information, see page 252). The mushrooms add selenium, and the bell pepper, antioxidants. You can also serve the quinoa mixture as a salad, at room temperature or chilled.

Serving Suggestions: For side dishes that will add more protein to the meal, try Edamame Succotash with Salsa (page 253), Sauteed Lima Beans and Spinach with Red Bell Pepper (page 239), or Tofu Fritters (page 250). For a crunchy salad, toss together a combination of thinly shredded red and green cabbage with a lemony mustard vinaigrette.

MAKES 6 SERVINGS
Prep: 15 minutes / Cook: about 30 minutes

> 2 tablespoons olive oil
>
> 1 red onion, quartered and thinly sliced
>
> 1 red bell pepper, cored, seeded, and cut into 2-inch-long thin strips
>
> 1 cup quinoa, rinsed very well and drained well
>
> 2 cups vegetable broth, homemade (page 101) or store-bought
>
> 10 ounces mushrooms, such as cremini, baby bella, or white button, cleaned, tough stems removed, and mushrooms sliced
>
> $\frac{3}{4}$ cup frozen peas, thawed
>
> 1 tablespoon dried oregano
>
> $\frac{3}{4}$ teaspoon salt
>
> $\frac{1}{4}$ teaspoon black pepper

1. In a large nonstick skillet, heat oil over medium heat. Add onion and red bell pepper and cook, stirring frequently, until softened, about 5 minutes.

2. Stir in quinoa and cook, stirring frequently, until lightly colored, 1 to 2 minutes. Stir in broth and mushrooms. Cover and simmer until broth is absorbed, about 25 minutes.

3. Stir in peas, oregano, salt, and pepper, gently heat through, and then serve.

Add-In: Stir 2 tablespoons grated Parmesan-style soy cheese into quinoa mixture along with peas in step 3.

Make-Ahead Tip: Quinoa mixture can be made up to two days ahead and refrigerated, tightly covered. To serve, spoon into nonstick saucepan and gently heat, stirring frequently and adding a little more vegetable broth if the mixture becomes too dry.

Pumpkin Polenta with Wild Mushroom Ragout

Orange-colored vegetables and squashes such as pumpkin are a great source of beta-carotene, an antioxidant. If you've never made polenta, this is a simple introduction—it does take a little cooking and stirring, but sometimes standing by the stove can be a peaceful activity. Usually polenta is made with just cornmeal and is prepared two ways: soft like a pudding or firm so it can be cut into squares or other shapes. This recipe shows you the latter method. Polenta can also be bought in a tube form and is usually in the refrigerator section near the produce or sometimes near the refrigerated pastas. If you make your own polenta, then you know exactly what's in it. You can substitute mashed, cooked butternut or hubbard squash, or canned solid-pack pumpkin puree for the cooked-from-scratch pumpkin. The mushroom ragout can double as a pasta sauce.

There are several steps in making this recipe, but the results are special, and the dish is perfect for company. It may help to know that the components can be made a day ahead.

Serving Suggestions: Round out the menu with Broccoli and Orange Salad with Water Chestnuts (page 118), Pan-Seared Broccoli and Garlic (page 234), Orange and Watercress Salad with Ginger-Mustard Dressing (page 125), a salad with dark leafy greens, or chilled, lightly cooked asparagus sprinkled with grated lemon zest or Gremolata (page 265).

MAKES 6 SERVINGS

Prep: 10 minutes / Soak: 30 minutes / Cook: about 50 minutes

Polenta:

1 cup yellow cornmeal

$3/4$ teaspoon salt

1 cup cooked, mashed pumpkin, well drained, fresh or canned

Mushroom Ragout:

2 teaspoons olive oil

1 large onion, finely chopped

4 ounces hot Italian-style meatless soy sausage links, thinly sliced

2 cloves garlic, finely chopped

$3/4$ pound wild or white button mushrooms, or a mixture, cleaned, tough stems removed, and mushrooms thinly sliced

$1/2$ cup dry white wine

$1\frac{1}{2}$ cups vegetable broth, homemade (page 101) or store-bought

$\frac{1}{2}$ teaspoon dried thyme, crumbled

$\frac{1}{4}$ teaspoon dried rosemary, crumbled

1 tablespoon all-purpose flour

$\frac{1}{4}$ cup finely chopped fresh parsley (optional)

Nonstick olive oil cooking spray

6 tablespoons grated Parmesan-syle soy cheese

1. For the polenta: In a large nonstick saucepan, stir together cornmeal and 2 cups of water. Set aside to soak for 30 minutes. Then stir in salt and another $1\frac{1}{2}$ cups of water. Heat to a simmer over medium heat, stirring constantly with a wooden spoon. Cook, stirring almost constantly, until mixture binds together and leaves sides of pan, about 15 minutes.

2. Stir in pumpkin until well blended and cook for 5 minutes longer, stirring often. Spread polenta evenly in an ungreased 13 x 9 x 2-inch baking dish. Set aside.

3. For the ragout: In a very large nonstick skillet, heat oil over medium heat. Add onion and cook, stirring occasionally, for 2 minutes. Add sausage and cook, stirring occasionally, for 2 minutes. Add garlic and cook for 1 minute. Stir in mushrooms and wine and cook, stirring occasionally, until mixture is almost dry, about 5 minutes. Stir in broth, thyme, and rosemary. Cover and simmer for 5 minutes.

4. In a small cup, stir together 2 tablespoons of water and flour until smooth. Stir into mushroom mixture in the skillet. Cover and simmer, stirring occasionally, until mushrooms are tender and sauce is slightly thickened, 5 to 10 minutes. Stir in parsley, if using.

5. Meanwhile, heat the broiler. Lightly coat a large broiler pan with cooking spray.

6. Turn polenta out onto a cutting board. Cut it lengthwise in half and cut each half crosswise into six equal rectangles. Transfer to the broiler pan.

7. Broil polenta 2 inches from heat until lightly browned on top, 1 to 2 minutes.

8. To serve, place a piece of polenta on each serving plate. Spoon half of the mushroom ragout over the polenta on the plates, then top with remaining polenta pieces. Cover with the remaining mushroom ragout, sprinkle with cheese, and serve at once.

Make-Ahead Tip: Both the polenta and the ragout can be made a day ahead and refrigerated. Bring the polenta to room temperature before broiling. Gently reheat the ragout in a saucepan, being careful not to let boil.

Spinach-Corn Couscous with Baked Tofu

When semolina or durum wheat is ground into a flour, it's used to make pasta, and when it's ground into granules, it becomes couscous. The instant version of couscous requires no real cooking, just a quick steep in boiling water or other liquid. Experiment with some of the different varieties of packaged baked tofu available in the supermarket or use cubed plain firm tofu and season the tofu mixture in step 2 with your favorite herbs or spices, such as cumin, curry, or thyme.

Serving Suggestions: Arrange a platter of bottled roasted red peppers and sliced tomatoes. Offer a bottle or cruet of balsamic vinegar for drizzling. Leftovers of the couscous dish, if any, can be all mixed together and served as a salad.

MAKES 6 SERVINGS
Prep: 10 minutes / Cook: 10 minutes

$1\frac{1}{2}$ cups whole-grain couscous

3 cups boiling water

2 tablespoons olive oil

2 packages (about 8 ounces each) baked tofu, any flavor, diced

$\frac{1}{2}$ cup chopped scallions

$\frac{1}{2}$ cup plus 1 tablespoon vegetable broth, homemade (page 101) or store-bought

1 bag (about 6 ounces) baby spinach, well rinsed

1 cup frozen corn kernels, thawed

1. In a heatproof bowl, cover couscous with the 3 cups boiling water. Let stand until water is absorbed, about 10 minutes. Fluff couscous with a fork. Stir in olive oil.

2. Meanwhile, in a medium-size nonstick skillet, combine tofu, scallions, and $\frac{1}{2}$ cup broth. Cook over medium-high heat, stirring frequently, until heated through, about 4 minutes.

3. At the same time, in a large nonstick skillet, combine spinach, corn, and the remaining tablespoon of vegetable broth. Cover and steam over medium-high heat until spinach is wilted and corn is heated through, about 1 minute. Remove to cutting board and coarsely chop spinach. Stir into couscous.

4. To serve, spoon tofu mixture over couscous.

Chili con Soy

Even though this chili tastes likes it contains ground beef, it doesn't—the secret is soy crumbles, with the added benefit of isoflavones. And the tomato sauce introduces lycopene.

Serving Suggestions: You can add all sorts of ingredients to this "meaty" chili mix before you serve up a bowlful. Some suggestions: corn kernels, kidney beans, black beans, or steamed cubes of butternut squash. Or use this basic chili to top a soy hot dog (page 78), a corn muffin, an acorn squash half, or a baked potato, white or sweet.

MAKES 4 SERVINGS (ABOUT 3½ CUPS)
Prep: 5 minutes / Cook: 30 minutes

> 1 tablespoon olive oil
> ½ small green bell pepper, cored, seeded, and chopped
> 1 package (14 ounces) ground beef-style soy protein
> ¼ teaspoon salt
> ⅛ teaspoon black pepper
> 1 cup Homemade All-Purpose Tomato Sauce (page 259) or bottled meatless marinara sauce
> 1 tablespoon chili powder
> 1 teaspoon ground cumin
> 2 teaspoons Dijon mustard
> 1 teaspoon Worcestershire sauce

1. In a large nonstick skillet, heat oil over medium heat. Add green pepper and cook, stirring occasionally, for 1 minute. Add soy, salt, and pepper, and cook, stirring frequently to break up, until soy is lightly colored, about 5 minutes.

2. Add tomato sauce, ½ cup water, chili powder, cumin, mustard, and Worcestershire, and simmer, stirring occasionally, for 20 minutes. Serve.

Make-Ahead Tip: Chili can be refrigerated for up to three days, or frozen for up to a month.

Black Bean and Tortilla Casserole with Salsa

Big flavor is what this casserole delivers, as well as lycopene and fiber (9 grams), and no saturated fat. To bump up the protein, add 12 ounces of firm tofu, cubed, to the zucchini mixture in step 2. The casserole is quick to assemble and feeds a small crowd. Leftovers make an easy snack, reheated in a microwave, toaster oven, or conventional oven.

Serving Suggestions: For other menu choices, try Edamame Succotash with Salsa (page 253) and Scalloped Corn with Sun-Dried Tomatoes (page 248). Keep a salad easy: red bell pepper and spinach, or avocado and orange.

MAKES 6 SERVINGS
Prep: 10 minutes / Cook: 20 minutes

Nonstick olive oil cooking spray

1 medium-size zucchini, trimmed, quartered lengthwise, and thinly sliced crosswise

3 cups bottled salsa, or a double recipe of Mexican Tomato Salsa with Serrano Chile (page 52)

1 can (19 ounces) black beans, drained and rinsed

1 cup chopped scallions (about 1 bunch)

1 teaspoon ground cumin

Twelve 6-inch corn tortillas, each torn into 5 or 6 pieces

2 cups (8 ounces) grated Monterey Jack–style or cheddar-style soy cheese

1. Heat oven to 400°F. Lightly coat a 13 x 9 x 2-inch baking dish with cooking spray.

2. In a medium-size bowl, stir together zucchini, salsa, black beans, scallions, and cumin.

3. In the prepared baking dish, layer half the tortilla pieces, half the bean mixture, and half the cheese. Repeat layering.

4. Bake until heated through and bubbling around edges, about 20 minutes. Let stand 10 minutes before serving.

Make-Ahead Tip: Casserole can be assembled earlier in the day, refrigerated, and then popped in the oven for about a half hour before serving.

Black Bean Chili with Chipotle

This is probably the fastest-to-fix chili you'll ever come across. What fools you into thinking it has simmered for hours is the smoky spiciness of the canned chipotle chiles, which add a depth of flavor. The stewed tomatoes are a good source of lycopene, and the beans provide protein and fiber. If you want an even richer flavor, stir in an ounce of grated bittersweet chocolate. For more protein and a "meatier" texture, add 4 ounces of firm tofu, cut into small cubes. For chili that includes soy "meat," see Chili con Soy (page 153).

Serving Suggestion: Top with shredded Monterey Jack–style soy cheese, and a scattering of crumbled Homemade Tortilla Chips (page 55) or store-bought baked low-fat tortilla chips. A good choice for a side dish is Edamame Succotash with Salsa (page 253). Or how about a combination of corn kernels and chopped bottled roasted red peppers heated together with a little vegetable broth and shredded pepper Jack–style soy cheese? For a crunchy go-with, toss shredded carrot with shredded jicama, drizzle with a little cider vinegar, and season with salt and pepper.

MAKES 4 SERVINGS

Prep: 10 minutes / Cook: 15 minutes

> 1 can (15 ounces) black beans, drained and rinsed
>
> 1 can (15 ounces) pinto or Roman beans, drained and rinsed
>
> 1 can (14.5 ounces) stewed tomatoes, sliced or chopped, with liquid
>
> 1 to 2 canned chipotle chiles in adobo sauce, or 2 fresh jalapeños, seeded and chopped, or 1 can (4 ounces) chopped jalapeños
>
> 1 teaspoon ground cumin
>
> $\frac{1}{2}$ teaspoon salt
>
> $\frac{1}{4}$ teaspoon ground cinnamon
>
> $\frac{1}{8}$ teaspoon ground cloves
>
> Plain soy yogurt, for garnish (optional)

In a large saucepan, stir together all the ingredients. Gently heat over medium heat, stirring occasionally, until heated through, about 15 minutes. Spoon into bowl and dollop with soy yogurt, if using.

Make-Ahead Tip: Chili can be refrigerated for up to three days or frozen for up to two months. The spiciness of the chili may intensify over time.

Fennel and Chickpea Stew with Apricots and Raisins

It may seem like there are a lot of ingredients in this dish, but a good number of them are spices and seasonings. The stew is an easy prep, and although the cooking is long, it takes care of itself in the oven. Fennel is a vegetable that resembles celery but has a delicate licorice or anise flavor. It is delicious raw and is also especially yummy when slowly cooked, as in this recipe. Fennel is rich in vitamins A and C and is a good source of fiber—it contributes to the 10 grams per serving in this dish. For extra protein, add 8 ounces of spicy Italian-style soy sausage links, sliced, or chorizo-style soy sausage, casing removed and "meat" crumbled, along with the garlic in step 2.

Serving Suggestions: Serve over whole-grain couscous or regular brown rice or brown basmati rice, and accompany with Broccoli and Orange Salad with Water Chestnuts (page 118) or orange segments tossed with sliced radishes and drizzled with rice vinegar. For a more substantial side dish, try Broccoli Rabe with Garlic and Parmesan Cheese (page 232), Steamed Sesame Spinach (page 243), or Sauteed Lima Beans and Spinach with Red Bell Pepper (page 239).

MAKES 4 SERVINGS

Prep: 10 minutes / Cook: about 1 hour and 10 minutes

2 fresh fennel bulbs

1 tablespoon olive oil

1 large sweet onion such as Vidalia, chopped

2 cloves garlic, finely chopped

1 teaspoon ground ginger

1 teaspoon ground cinnamon

1 teaspoon ground nutmeg

$\frac{1}{2}$ teaspoon salt

$\frac{1}{4}$ teaspoon black pepper

$\frac{1}{4}$ cup golden raisins

$\frac{1}{4}$ cup dried pitted apricots, chopped

2 bay leaves

1 cup dry white wine or vegetable broth, homemade (page 101) or store-bought

1 pound ripe tomatoes, cored, seeded, and chopped, or 1 can (14.5 ounces) diced tomatoes

1 can (15 ounces) chickpeas, drained and rinsed

1. Trim stalks from fennel bulbs and reserve for other uses such as salad or soup making. Cut bulbs in half through the core and remove core. Cut halves into $\frac{1}{2}$-inch-thick wedges. Set aside.

2. In a large ovenproof pot, heat oil over medium heat. Add onion and cook until softened and lightly golden, about 8 minutes, stirring in garlic for the last 2 minutes of cooking.

3. Heat oven to 375°F.

4. Stir ginger, cinnamon, nutmeg, salt, and pepper into onion mixture, and cook, stirring frequently, for 1 minute. Stir in raisins, apricots, bay leaves, and white wine, and cook until wine is reduced by about half. Stir in fennel, tomato, and chickpeas. Cover pot and bring to a boil.

5. Place pot in 375 F. oven and cook until fennel is very tender, about 1 hour.

Make-Ahead Tip: Stew can be refrigerated for up to three days, or frozen for up to a month. Gently reheat it on the stove, stirring occasionally, adding a little vegetable broth or water if the stew appears too dry.

Nutty Lentil Loaf with Veggies and Mozzarella Cheese

Although this recipe takes some time to put together, the effort is well worth it. The result is a delicious loaf, full of mushrooms, carrots, red bell pepper, and Brazil nuts, that can be served warm, at room temperature, or even chilled. The bulghur and lentils combine to provide a hefty amount of protein, 19 grams per serving, and with no animal fat in sight. There are also 11 grams of fiber.

Serving Suggestions: Serve with cooked sweet potatoes mashed with soy milk, and sugar snap peas or a green salad. Leftover slices make very good sandwiches on whole-grain toast, with a little ketchup or mustard or both, or soy mayonnaise. Or arrange slices on a bed of dark leafy greens for a salad.

MAKES 8 SERVINGS

Prep: 30 minutes / Stand: 25 minutes / Cook: 1 hour

$1\frac{1}{2}$ cups boiling water

$\frac{1}{2}$ cup bulghur

1 tablespoon olive oil

1 medium-size sweet onion such as Vidalia, chopped

10 ounces fresh button mushrooms, cleaned, tough stems removed, and mushrooms coarsely chopped

1 red bell pepper, cored, seeded, and chopped

1 medium-size carrot, trimmed, peeled, and grated

3 cloves garlic, finely chopped

$\frac{1}{2}$ teaspoon salt

Nonstick olive oil cooking spray

3 cups canned brown lentils or cooked dried lentils

$1\frac{1}{2}$ cups fresh whole-wheat bread crumbs (2 slices)

$\frac{3}{4}$ cup Brazil nuts or pecans, ground

6 ounces ($1\frac{1}{2}$ cups) mozzarella-style soy cheese, shredded

$\frac{1}{2}$ cup liquid egg substitute

2 tablespoons Worcestershire sauce

$\frac{1}{4}$ cup plus 2 tablespoons Dijon mustard

$\frac{1}{4}$ teaspoon black pepper

1 cup ketchup

1. In a small bowl, pour the boiling water over bulghur. Let stand 25 minutes. Drain in a sieve.

2. In a large nonstick skillet, heat oil over medium heat. Add onion and cook, stirring occasionally, until golden brown, about 8 minutes. Add mushrooms and bell pepper, and cook, stirring occasionally, until mushrooms release liquid, about 4 minutes. Increase heat to medium-high and cook until mixture is dry, about 8 minutes. Stir in carrot, garlic, and ¼ teaspoon of the salt, and cook, stirring occasionally, for 2 minutes. Scrape mixture onto plate.

3. Heat oven to 375°F. Line a 9 x 5 x 3-inch loaf pan with foil. Lightly coat foil with cooking spray.

4. In a large bowl, mash 2 cups of the lentils with a potato masher. Add remaining lentils, bulghur, bread crumbs, nuts, cheese, egg substitute, Worcestershire sauce, 2 tablespoons mustard, black pepper, vegetable mixture, and the remaining ¼ teaspoon salt. Mix together with clean hands or a spoon until well blended. Turn mixture into prepared pan and press to pack.

5. Bake for 1 hour, then let stand for 10 minutes. Taking hold of the foil, lift loaf out of the pan onto a cutting board. Let stand for 15 minutes.

6. In a small saucepan, combine ketchup and ¼ cup mustard and gently heat, stirring occasionally, to make a sauce.

7. Remove the foil from sides of loaf. Using a serrated knife, carefully cut loaf into 1-inch-thick slices (they will be crumbly). Serve with sauce.

Make-Ahead Tip: Uncooked loaf can be refrigerated up to a day. Cooked loaf can be refrigerated up to three days, or frozen up to a month. Slice the loaf before freezing. Reheat slices in microwave or 350°F oven.

Chickpea and Spinach Loaf with Mustard-Ketchup Topping

This loaf has a lot going for it—fiber, antioxidants, nonanimal protein, and isoflavones. And as with most loaves, sliced leftovers can be the beginning of very tasty sandwiches.

Serving Suggestions: To round out a menu, mash cooked sweet potatoes with unsweetened soy milk and a little maple syrup, and grill or boil some corn on the cob, or simmer corn kernels with chopped pickled jalapeños.

MAKES 6 SERVINGS

Prep: 20 minutes / Cook: about 1 hour

    2 teaspoons olive oil
    1 small onion, finely chopped
    1 bag (about 6 ounces) baby spinach
    1 medium-size carrot, trimmed, peeled, and shredded
    3 cloves garlic, minced or crushed through a press
    $\frac{3}{4}$ teaspoon dried Italian seasoning
    $\frac{1}{2}$ teaspoon salt
    $\frac{1}{4}$ teaspoon black pepper
    Nonstick olive oil cooking spray
    7 ounces ($\frac{1}{2}$ of 14-ounce cake) firm tofu, drained and blotted dry with paper towels
    1 can (15 ounces) chickpeas, rinsed and drained
    1 cup cooked brown rice (see Note below)
    $\frac{3}{4}$ cup fresh whole-wheat bread crumbs (about 1 slice)
    1 large egg white
    $\frac{1}{2}$ cup ketchup
    1 tablespoon Dijon mustard

1. In a large nonstick skillet, heat oil over medium heat. Add onion and cook, stirring frequently, until softened, about 5 minutes. Increase heat to medium-high and stir in spinach, carrot, garlic, Italian seasoning, salt, and pepper. Cook, stirring constantly, until spinach wilts, about 3 minutes. Set aside to cool slightly.

2. Heat oven to 375°F. Line a rimmed baking sheet with foil. Lightly coat foil with cooking spray.

3. In a large bowl, mash together tofu and chickpeas with a potato masher. Add spinach mixture, rice, bread crumbs, egg white, 2 tablespoons of the ketchup and $1\frac{1}{2}$ teaspoons of the mustard. Mix with a spoon or clean hands until well blended. Let stand for 5 minutes. In a small bowl, stir together the remaining ketchup and mustard.

4. Shape loaf mixture into a 7 x 3$\frac{1}{2}$-inch loaf on the center of a prepared baking sheet. Spread ketchup mixture over loaf.

5. Bake until browned, 50 to 55 minutes. Let stand for 10 minutes before cutting into thick slices with a serrated knife.

Make-Ahead Tip: Uncooked loaf can be refrigerated for a day. Cooked loaf can be refrigerated for up to three days or frozen for up to a month. Slice the cooked loaf before freezing. Reheat slices in microwave or 350°F oven.

Note: If you have no leftover cooked brown rice, simmer $\frac{1}{3}$ cup brown rice with 1 cup water in a covered saucepan until rice is tender and water is absorbed, about 45 minutes. Let cool before using.

Spinach Enchiladas with Jack Cheese and Soybeans

Spinach and cabbage together pack a bundle of suspected compounds thought to fight cancer, and if you use the soybeans, there is the added benefit of isoflavones and additional protein. Experiment with some of the different flavored low-fat tortillas.

Serving Suggestions: Slice a ripe avocado and drizzle with orange juice vinaigrette.

MAKES 4–8 SERVINGS (1–2 ENCHILADAS PER SERVING)
Prep: 15 minutes / Cook: about 40 minutes

Nonstick olive oil cooking spray

$\frac{1}{4}$ head Savoy cabbage, shredded

1 pound fresh spinach, washed, tough stems removed, and drained

1 can (about 15 ounces) organic yellow soybeans, or pinto beans, drained and rinsed

1 cup frozen corn kernels, thawed

1 fresh jalapeño, seeded and chopped, or 1 canned chipotle chile in adobo, chopped

1 teaspoon chili powder

$\frac{1}{2}$ teaspoon salt

$\frac{1}{4}$ teaspoon black pepper

Eight 8-inch low-fat flour tortillas

3 cups bottled salsa, or a double recipe of Mexican Tomato Salsa with Serrano Chile (page 52)

1 cup (4 ounces) shredded Jack-style or cheddar-style soy cheese

1. Heat oven to 400°F. Coat a 13 x 9 x 2-inch baking dish with nonstick cooking spray.

2. Coat a large skillet with nonstick cooking spray. Heat over medium-high heat. Add cabbage and cook, stirring frequently, until it begins to wilt and color around edges, about 6 minutes. Stir in spinach and lower heat. Cover the skillet and cook until spinach wilts, 1 to 2 minutes. Remove from heat.

3. Stir beans, corn, chili powder, salt, and pepper into spinach mixture.

4. Coat a medium-size nonstick skillet with nonstick cooking spray. Heat it over medium heat. Place 1 tortilla in the skillet and heat until softened, about 30 seconds. Turn over and warm the other side for about 15 seconds. Remove tortilla to a work surface. Spoon $\frac{1}{2}$ cup spinach mixture down the center of the warmed tortilla and roll it up. Place tortilla, seam side down, in the prepared baking dish. Repeat with remaining filling and tortillas.

5. Spoon salsa over enchiladas. Cover the baking dish with aluminum foil.

6. Bake until heated through, about 20 minutes.

7. Uncover baking dish and sprinkle top with cheese. Return the dish to the oven and bake until cheese is melted, 3 to 5 minutes.

Make-Ahead Tip: Filling mixture can be refrigerated for up to a day. The casserole can be assembled a day ahead and refrigerated. Leftover enchiladas can be rewarmed in a microwave or 350°F oven.

Southwest Lasagna with Spinach and Pinto Beans

Corn tortillas replace the lasagna noodles in this easy make-ahead dish.

Serving Suggestions: Toss together fresh or thawed frozen corn kernels, halved cherry tomatoes, and chopped fresh cilantro or parsley with Balsamic Vinaigrette (page 141).

MAKES 4 SERVINGS

Prep: 15 minutes / Cook: 40 minutes.

> Nonstick olive oil cooking spray
>
> 1 cup fresh cilantro leaves or fresh flat-leaf parsley leaves
>
> 1 small bunch scallions, trimmed and coarsely chopped
>
> $\frac{1}{4}$ teaspoon salt
>
> $\frac{1}{4}$ teaspoon black pepper
>
> 1 package (about 10 ounces) fresh baby spinach
>
> 1 can (15 ounces) pinto beans, drained and rinsed
>
> 1 cup bottled salsa
>
> $\frac{1}{2}$ teaspoon ground cumin
>
> Eight 6-inch corn tortillas
>
> 8 ounces (about 2 cups) Monterey pepper Jack–style soy cheese, shredded, or 1
>   package (8 ounces) preshredded Monterey Jack–style soy cheese blend

1. Heat oven to 425°F. Lightly coat an 8 x 8 x 2-inch square baking dish with cooking spray.

2. In a large food processor (or with a knife and a cutting board), use on-and-off pulses to chop together cilantro, scallions, salt, and pepper until coarsely chopped. Add spinach a handful or two at a time and pulse until coarsely chopped. (If mixture starts to become a puree at the bottom of the processor, scrape the mixture into a bowl before continuing to chop the spinach.)

3. In a small bowl, stir together pinto beans, salsa, and cumin.

4. In the bottom of a baking dish, arrange 4 tortillas, overlapping. Cover with half of the bean mixture, half of the spinach mixture, and half of the cheese. Top with remaining 4 tortillas, bean mixture, spinach mixture, and cheese. Gently press down layers to compact. Cover the baking dish with aluminum foil.

5. Bake until heated through and bubbly, about 25 minutes. Uncover. Continue baking until cheese on top is golden, about 15 minutes. Let cool for 10 minutes before serving.

Make-Ahead Tip: Lasagna can be assembled a day ahead and refrigerated (uncooked). Increase the baking time by 5 to 10 minutes if you transfer the lasagna directly from refrigerator to oven. Leftovers can be refrigerated for up to three days and reheated in a 350°F oven or microwave.

Chickpeas with Squas

Feta-style soy cheese— ...es in the refrigerated
health food section ... as well as isoflavones to this
Mediterranean r ... in the tomatoes. When the
dish comes o ... .quid in the bottom, but this will
gradually be a.

Serving Suggestions. ... or brown basmati rice and add a salad of
thinly sliced fresh fennei ... .d with chopped toasted Brazil nuts and
splashed with a little balsamic ... e vinegar. For another side dish, add Pan-Seared
Broccoli and Garlic (page 234)— ...ne broccoli or substitute cauliflower. The cold
chickpea leftovers are delicious as a salad.

MAKES 6 SERVINGS

Prep: 15 minutes / Cook: 55 minutes

    Nonstick olive oil cooking spray

    1 can (29 ounces) chickpeas, drained and rinsed, or $3\frac{1}{2}$ cups

    $\frac{3}{4}$ cup crumbled feta-style soy cheese

    2 teaspoons Dijon mustard

    1 can (14.5 ounces) diced tomatoes, drained

    $\frac{1}{4}$ teaspoon salt

    $\frac{1}{4}$ teaspoon black pepper

    2 tablespoons olive oil

    1 onion, coarsely chopped

    1 red bell pepper, cored, seeded, and coarsely chopped

    2 teaspoons dried marjoram

    2 cloves garlic, finely chopped

    1 large yellow summer squash, trimmed, halved lengthwise, or quartered if very large, then cut crosswise into chunks

    1 large zucchini, trimmed, halved lengthwise, or quartered if very large, then cut crosswise into chunks

1. Heat oven to 375°F. Lightly coat an 8 x 8 x 2-inch baking dish with cooking spray.

2. In the baking dish, stir together chickpeas, cheese, mustard, half of the tomatoes, salt, and pepper.

3. In a large nonstick skillet, heat 1 tablespoon of the oil over medium heat. Add onion, bell pepper, and marjoram and cook, stirring occasionally, until onion and bell pepper are slightly softened, about 5 minutes. Add garlic and cook 1 minute. Stir into bean mixture in the baking dish.

4. In the same skillet, heat the remaining oil. Add squash and zucchini and cook, stirring occasionally, until slightly softened, about 5 minutes. Stir in the remaining tomato. Spoon over bean mixture in the baking dish. Cover the dish with aluminum foil.

5. Bake until bubbly and heated through, about 45 minutes. Let stand for 10 minutes before serving.

Make-Ahead Tip: Casserole can be assembled earlier in day and refrigerated. If transferring it directly from refrigerator to oven, increase the baking time. Leftovers can be refrigerated for up to three days, and are easily reheated in a microwave or conventional oven at 350°F.

Red Lentil and Sweet Potato Stew with Indian Spices

Spiced with coriander, cumin, turmeric, and ginger, this stew is thick and creamy, similar to an Indian dal, and textured with small pieces of sweet potato, which is rich in beta-carotene, a powerful antioxidant.

Serving Suggestions: Spoon over brown basmati, regular brown, or red Butan rice and sprinkle with chopped fresh cilantro or parsley. For side-dish add-ons, try Stewed Fennel with Carrots and Orange (page 244), Edamame Succotash with Salsa (page 253), or create a fruit salad with diced papaya, watermelon, cantaloupe, mango, and strawberries to temper the spicy heat of the stew as well as up the antioxidant quotient. You can also serve the lentils as a side dish with broiled fish, such as Halibut with Orange–Ginger Sauce (page 199) or Broiled Salmon with Cumin and Lemon (page 192).

MAKES 6 SERVINGS

Prep: 10 minutes / Cook: 50 minutes

> 2 tablespoons olive oil
>
> 1 medium-size onion, finely chopped
>
> 1 medium-size sweet potato, peeled and cut into $\frac{1}{8}$-inch dice
>
> 1 tablespoon peeled, finely chopped fresh ginger
>
> 2 cloves garlic, finely chopped
>
> 1 cup dried red lentils, picked over and rinsed
>
> 2 teaspoons ground coriander
>
> 2 teaspoons ground cumin
>
> 1 teaspoon ground turmeric
>
> 1 teaspoon ground ginger
>
> $\frac{1}{2}$ teaspoon crushed red pepper flakes
>
> 1 can (14.5 ounces) diced tomatoes
>
> 4 cups water, or 2 cups water plus 2 cups vegetable broth, homemade (page 101) or store-bought
>
> $\frac{1}{2}$ teaspoon salt

1. In a large nonstick saucepan, heat oil over medium heat. Add onion and cook, stirring occasionally, until softened, about 5 minutes. Add sweet potato and cook, stirring occasionally, until crisp-tender, about 5 minutes. Reduce heat to low.

2. Stir in fresh ginger and garlic. Stir in lentils, coriander, cumin, turmeric, ground ginger, and pepper flakes until well combined. Add tomatoes and water or water-broth combination. Bring to a boil. Lower heat and simmer until potatoes and lentils are softened, about 30 minutes.

3. Stir in salt and simmer another 10 minutes to blend flavors. Stir or whisk to break up potatoes and lentils and thicken the stew.

Make-Ahead Tip: Stew can be refrigerated for up to three days.

Beans and Franks with Molasses

Here's a meatless variation of an American classic—it's full of beneficial lyocpene from the ketchup and isoflavones from the soybeans and soy franks. After tasting a variety of vegetarian baked beans, I like Bush's brand best. But try your own taste test and decide for yourself.

Serving Suggestions: To continue with the American classic theme, spoon a little Thousand Island Dressing (page 138) over a wedge of iceberg lettuce or some dark, leafy greens tossed with cherry or small pear tomatoes.

MAKES 6 SERVINGS
Prep: 5 minutes / Cook: 12 minutes

> 1 can (16 ounces) vegetarian baked beans, not drained
> 1 can (16 ounces) organic yellow soybeans, not drained
> 3 tablespoons ketchup
> 2 tablespoons molasses
> 1 teaspoon Worcestershire sauce
> $\frac{1}{4}$ teaspoon salt
> 1 package (12 ounces) soy hot dogs, cut into $\frac{1}{2}$-inch pieces

1. In a medium-size saucepan, stir together baked beans, soybeans, ketchup, molasses, Worcestershire, and salt. Simmer for 10 minutes
2. Add hot dogs and heat through, about 2 minutes.

Make-Ahead Tip: Dish can be refrigerated for up to three days.

Smoky Cheese Enchiladas

It's the green olive topping that really makes this dish special. You can substitute any melting soy cheese, such as Monterey Jack–style or queso blanco–style, for the smoked cheddar, if you prefer a different flavor. For extra texture, reduce the tofu to six ounces and add a half cup of black beans to the filling mix. If you'd like extra sauce for serving, heat a second can of enchilada sauce.

Serving Suggestions: Two salad choices here: sliced avocado with orange slices drizzled with Honey-Cilantro Vinaigrette (minus the soy sauce, page 136), or matchsticks of jicama or sliced radishes and halved cherry tomatoes, tossed with a citrusy vinaigrette.

MAKES 4–8 SERVINGS
Prep: 20 minutes / Cook: 30 minutes

> 1 package (12.3 ounces) silken firm tofu, drained and blotted dry with paper towels
>
> 3 cups (12 ounces) shredded smoked cheddar–style soy cheese
>
> 4 scallions, trimmed and finely chopped (white and green parts separated)
>
> $\frac{1}{4}$ cup finely chopped fresh cilantro
>
> 1 tablespoon chopped canned green chiles
>
> 1 can (10 ounces) enchilada sauce
>
> Eight 6-inch corn tortillas
>
> 1 large ripe tomato, cored and finely chopped
>
> 12 green olives, pitted and finely chopped

1. Heat oven to 350°F.

2. In a medium-size bowl, mash tofu. Stir in half of the soy cheese, the white part of the scallions, 2 tablespoons of the cilantro, and the green chiles.

3. In a small skillet, heat enchilada sauce over medium heat. One at a time, dip tortillas into sauce to soften and place on a waxed paper–lined work surface. Top with $\frac{1}{3}$ cup tofu-cheese mixture. Roll up and place, seam-side down, in a 9 x 6 x 2-inch baking dish. Repeat with remaining tortillas and filling. Pour remaining enchilada sauce from skillet evenly over enchiladas.

4. Bake, uncovered, until hot and bubbly, about 25 minutes. Sprinkle top evenly with the remaining cheese. Bake until cheese is melted, about 5 minutes. Remove from oven and garnish with tomato, olives, the green parts of the scallions, and the remaining cilantro.

Make-Ahead Tip: Enchiladas can be assembled in the baking dish earlier in the day and refrigerated, tightly covered. Leftovers can be rewarmed in a microwave or 350°F. oven.

Pomegranate-Glazed Tofu with Broccoli and Baby Corn

Now this is an unusual dish but very tasty. The pomegranate has been touted as possessing prostate cancer-fighting properties, and in this recipe, pomegranate syrup flavors the sauce. You can probably find the syrup in health food stores or the international food section of the supermarket—if not, substitute orange juice concentrate. And if you've never tried the prepackaged baked tofu, located in the refrigerator case of the produce section of the supermarket, then here's an introduction. This dish is best devoured immediately after cooking.

Serving Suggestions: Spoon over any grain, such as regular brown rice or brown basmati rice, or over rice noodles. Or, eat as is, with a shredded baby bok choy salad.

MAKES 4 SERVINGS
Prep: 10 minutes / Cook: 8 minutes

Sauce:

2 tablespoons cornstarch

$\frac{1}{4}$ cup cold water

2 tablespoons reduced-sodium soy sauce

1 tablespoon pomegranate syrup or orange juice concentrate

1 tablespoon rice vinegar

2 teaspoons dark sesame oil

1 teaspoon peeled, finely chopped fresh ginger

Vegetables:

1 tablespoon light olive oil

2 tablespoons vegetable broth, homemade (page 101) or store-bought

2 large broccoli crowns, cut into small pieces

2 cloves garlic, finely chopped

1 red bell pepper, cored, seeded, and cut into thin strips

1 can (15 ounces) baby corn, drained and rinsed

2 packages (about 8 ounces each) baked tofu (your choice of flavor), cut into narrow strips, or 1 pound Susan's Marinated Five-Spice Tofu (page 65)

1. For the sauce: In a small bowl, stir together cornstarch and the $\frac{1}{4}$ cup cold water until smooth. Stir in soy sauce, pomegranate syrup, vinegar, sesame oil, and ginger.

2. For the vegetables: In a large nonstick skillet or wok, heat together oil and vegetable broth over medium heat. Add broccoli and garlic. Cover and cook until broccoli is crisp-tender, about 3 minutes. Stir in bell pepper, baby corn, and tofu, and cook, stirring frequently, for 2 minutes. Pour in the sauce and cook, stirring frequently, until sauce is thickened and mixture is heated through, 1 to 2 minutes. Serve immediately.

Thai-Style Sweet and Sour Tofu with Vegetables

If you've never worked with tofu in a main dish, here's an easy recipe that demonstrates some of its qualities. Remember that tofu has a very subtle flavor, some may even say bland. With all the vegetables and seasonings in this stir-fry, it becomes a background ingredient, contributing a "meaty" texture, as well as nonanimal protein and isoflavones. Once you've assembled the ingredients, the stir-fry takes just a few minutes to cook.

Serving Suggestions: To soak up the sauce, rice is the perfect accompaniment—jasmine, brown basmati, or brown rice are all good choices.

MAKES 4 SERVINGS
Prep: 15 minutes / Cook: 6 minutes

$\frac{1}{2}$ cup vegetable broth, homemade (page 101) or store-bought

$\frac{1}{4}$ cup freshly squeezed lime juice (about 4 limes)

2 tablespoons soy sauce

2 teaspoons organic sugar (evaporated cane juice)

2 teaspoons cornstarch

1 tablespoon olive oil

4 cloves garlic, finely chopped

1 tablespoon finely chopped, peeled fresh ginger

2 fresh serrano or other hot chiles, cored, seeded, and finely chopped

1 red bell pepper, cored, seeded, and cut into $\frac{1}{2}$-inch squares

4 scallions, trimmed and thinly sliced

1 medium-size zucchini, trimmed, cut lengthwise into quarters, and then crosswise into $\frac{1}{4}$-inch-thick pieces

12 canned baby corn, rinsed

$\frac{1}{4}$ pound Napa cabbage, cut into thin shreds

1 pound firm tofu, drained, blotted dry with paper towels, and cut into $\frac{1}{2}$-inch cubes

1. In a small bowl, whisk together broth, lime juice, soy sauce, sugar, and cornstarch until smooth.

2. In a large nonstick skillet or wok with a lid, heat 2 teaspoons of the oil over medium-high heat. Add garlic, ginger, and chiles and cook, stirring, for 30 seconds. Add to broth mixture.

3. Heat the remaining oil in the skillet. Add bell pepper, scallions, and zucchini and cook, stirring, until crisp-tender, 2 to 3 minutes. Add baby corn and cabbage and cook, stirring, for 1 minute. Add tofu and broth mixture. Cover and simmer until cabbage is just wilted, tofu is heated through, and sauce is lightly thickened, 1 to 2 minutes. Serve at once.

Make-Ahead Tip: All the vegetables and the tofu can be prepared earlier in the day and refrigerated. Let come to room temperature before cooking so the chilly ingredients don't increase the cooking time.

Apple and Sausage Skillet Dish with Sweet Potatoes and Cheddar Cheese

Sweet potatoes are a source of antioxidants, and the soy sausage and soy cheddar cheese have beneficial isoflavones.

Serving Suggestions: Broccoli and Orange Salad with Water Chestnuts (page 118) boosts the nutritional value of this meal even more, or toss together spinach and orange segments, sprinkle with a citrus vinaigrette, and garnish with toasted sliced almonds.

MAKES 4 SERVINGS

Prep: 15 minutes / Cook: about 15 minutes

1 pound sweet potatoes, peeled and cut into $\frac{1}{2}$-inch cubes

2 tablespoons light olive oil

1 sweet onion such as Vidalia, diced

1 small red bell pepper, cored, seeded, and cut into thin 2-inch-long strips

1 Granny Smith apple, with skin on, cored and thinly sliced

$\frac{1}{2}$ cup apple or orange juice

Nonstick olive oil cooking spray

1 package (8 ounces) soy sausage links, sliced $\frac{1}{4}$-inch thick

$\frac{1}{4}$ teaspoon salt

$\frac{1}{4}$ teaspoon black pepper

$\frac{1}{4}$ cup shredded cheddar-style soy cheese

1. In a large saucepan of boiling water, cook sweet potato just until firm–tender, about 5 minutes. Drain.

2. In a large nonstick skillet, heat oil over medium heat. Add onion and bell pepper and cook, stirring occasionally, until onion and pepper are slightly softened, about 4 minutes.

3. Add apple slices, sweet potato, and apple juice to the skillet and cook, gently stirring occasionally, until apples are slightly softened, about 4 minutes.

4. Meanwhile, lightly coat a separate skillet with cooking spray and heat over medium heat. Add sausages and cook, stirring occasionally, until browned, about 4 minutes.

5. Gently stir sausages, salt, and pepper into apple mixture. Sprinkle with cheese, let melt slightly, and serve.

Make-Ahead Tip: Dish can be refrigerated for up to three days and gently reheated in a skillet.

Stir-Fried Cabbage with Spicy Sausage and Ginger

Inspired by a classic Chinese dish, this quick stir-fry makes good use of flavorful soy sausage, as well as phytonutrient-rich cabbage, an important cruciferous vegetable.

Serving Suggestions: In a second skillet, quickly stir-fry snow peas and cherry tomatoes in a little light olive oil; season with salt and pepper.

MAKES 4 SERVINGS
Prep: 10 minutes / Cook: about 12 minutes

  2 tablespoons light olive oil
  1 sweet onion such as Vidalia, finely chopped
  2 cloves garlic, finely chopped
  1 package (14 ounces) Italian-style soy sausage links, cut into thin slices
  $\frac{1}{2}$ small head green cabbage, coarsely shredded
  2 tablespoons peeled, finely chopped fresh ginger
  $\frac{1}{4}$ cup reduced-sodium soy sauce
  1 tablespoon dark sesame oil

1. In a large nonstick skillet, heat oil over medium-high heat. Add onion and cook, stirring occasionally, until softened, about 5 minutes. Add garlic and cook for 1 minute. Add sausage and cook, stirring occasionally, for 2 minutes to heat through.
2. Add cabbage, ginger, and soy sauce and cook, stirring occasionally, until cabbage is wilted and mixture is heated through, 2 to 4 minutes, depending on how crisp you like the cabbage. Stir in sesame oil and serve immediately.

Make-Ahead Tip: Cabbage mixture can be refrigerated for up to a day and gently reheated.

Herbed and Parmesan "Meatballs" in Tomato Sauce

There are vegetarian meatballs available in the supermarket, but if you make your own, then you know exactly what's in them and you can control the seasoning to your own taste. You can also make multiple batches of these and store them in the freezer to have on hand.

Serving Suggestions: Serve with a green salad with tomatoes and crusty garlic bread, or over whole-wheat spaghetti, or on a crusty roll with a melted nondairy cheese (page 74).

MAKES 4 TO 6 SERVINGS
Prep: 20 minutes / Cook: 15 minutes

    1 package (14 ounces) ground beef–style soy mixture

    1 large egg white

    $\frac{1}{4}$ cup grated onion

    $\frac{1}{4}$ cup grated Parmesan-style soy cheese

    $\frac{1}{4}$ cup chopped fresh parsley

    3 tablespoons olive oil

    2 cloves garlic, very finely chopped

    $\frac{1}{4}$ teaspoon salt

    2 teaspoons dried marjoram, basil, or Italian seasoning mix

    $\frac{1}{2}$ teaspoon fennel seeds, crushed (optional)

    $\frac{1}{4}$ cup fine dried bread crumbs or fresh bread crumbs

    1 recipe Fresh Tomato Sauce (page 258), or Homemade All-Purpose Tomato Sauce
       (page 259), or 1 jar (26 ounces) meatless marinara sauce

1. In a large bowl, combine soy mixture, egg white, onion, cheese, parsley, 1 tablespoon of the olive oil, garlic, salt, marjoram, and fennel seeds, if using. Gently mix together.

2. Gently shape mixture into twenty-four 1-inch balls. Roll balls in bread crumbs.

3. In a very large nonstick skillet, heat the remaining 2 tablespoons olive oil over medium heat. Add balls, in batches, and cook until browned on all sides, 1 to 2 minutes.

4. Meanwhile, in a large saucepan, heat tomato sauce over medium heat to a simmer. Transfer balls to sauce and simmer gently for 10 minutes before serving.

Make-Ahead Tip: Uncooked "meatballs" rolled in the bread crumbs can be refrigerated for up to a day, or frozen for up to a month. They can be cooked straight from the freezer as instructed in step 3, but increase the time to 4 to 5 minutes.

Three-Mushroom Stroganoff with Thyme

Instead of using heavy cream, this recipe substitutes pureed silken tofu to duplicate the creaminess of classic stroganoff, but without the saturated fat.

Serving Suggestions: Spoon the mushroom mixture over whole-wheat pasta, brown basmati rice, or whole-wheat toast points. Steamed carrots, broccoli florets, or Brussels sprouts tossed with a little olive oil and a dried herb such as oregano or marjoram round out the menu.

MAKES 8 SERVINGS
Prep: 20 minutes / Cook: 15 minutes

2 tablespoons light olive oil

1 sweet onion such as Vidalia, chopped

1 pound white button mushrooms, cleaned, tough stems removed, and mushrooms sliced

6 ounces portobello mushroom caps, cleaned and caps sliced

6 ounces cremini mushrooms, cleaned, tough stems removed, and mushrooms sliced

$\frac{1}{2}$ cup vegetable broth, homemade (page 101) or store-bought

1 box (12.3 ounces) silken soft tofu

2 tablespoons Dijon mustard

1 tablespoon freshly squeezed lemon juice

1 teaspoon dried thyme

$\frac{1}{2}$ teaspoon salt

$\frac{1}{4}$ teaspoon black pepper

$\frac{1}{4}$ cup finely chopped fresh parsley (optional)

1. In a large nonstick skillet, heat oil over medium heat. Add onion and cook, stirring occasionally, until softened, about 5 minutes. Add all the mushrooms and broth, stirring to mix well, cover, and bring to a gentle boil. Lower heat and simmer, covered, until mushrooms are tender, about 10 minutes.

2. While mushrooms are simmering, in a blender or small food processor, puree tofu.

3. Into mushrooms, stir mustard, lemon juice, thyme, salt, and pepper. Stir in pureed tofu until thoroughly combined and gently heat through, being careful not to let boil. Remove skillet from heat and stir in parsley if using. Serve over noodles, pasta, rice, or toast points.

Make-Ahead Tip: Mixture, without the parsley added, can be made a day ahead and refrigerated. Gently reheat in a large nonstick saucepan—do not let boil.

Mac and Three Cheeses with Scallion and Tomato

Thanks to the combination of soy cheeses and soy milk, this very rich, very tasty macaroni and cheese has only 1 gram of saturated fat. For a spicy variation, add a canned chipotle chile in adobo, seeded and chopped, or half a teaspoon crushed red pepper flakes along with the cheeses in step 3. Experiment with whole-wheat pasta shapes, such as rigatoni or rotelle.

Serving Suggestions: Toss small raw or blanched broccoli florets and bottled roasted red pepper strips with a little balsamic vinegar for a quick-fix salad.

MAKES 6 SERVINGS
Prep: 15 minutes / Cook: about 30 minutes

    10 ounces elbow macaroni
    1 can (14.5 ounces) diced tomatoes, drained
    1 cup chopped scallions (about 1 bunch)
    2 tablespoons olive oil
    $\frac{1}{4}$ teaspoon salt
    $\frac{1}{4}$ teaspoon black pepper
    Nonstick olive oil cooking spray
    3 tablespoons all-purpose flour
    $1\frac{1}{2}$ cups unsweetened soy milk
    $1\frac{1}{2}$ cups (6 ounces) shredded cheddar-style soy cheese
    $\frac{1}{2}$ cup (2 ounces) shredded pepper Jack–style soy cheese
    4 tablespoons grated Parmesan-style soy cheese
    $\frac{1}{2}$ cup fresh whole-wheat bread crumbs

1. In a large pot of lightly salted boiling water, cook macaroni according to package directions. Drain and return macaroni to pot. Stir in tomatoes, scallions, oil, salt, and pepper.

2. Heat oven to 400°F. Lightly coat a 2-quart baking dish with cooking spray.

3. In a medium-size nonstick saucepan, stir together flour and $\frac{1}{2}$ cup of the soy milk until smooth. Stir in the remaining soy milk, cheddar, pepper Jack, and 2 tablespoons of the Parmesan. Bring to a gentle simmer over medium heat, stirring occasionally. Continue cooking, stirring frequently, until cheeses are melted and sauce thickens, about another 3 minutes. Add to macaroni and stir to combine well. Scrape into the prepared baking dish.

4. In a small bowl, stir together the remaining 2 tablespoons Parmesan and the bread crumbs. Sprinkle evenly over macaroni mixture.

5. Bake until bubbly and top is lightly browned and crisped, 20 to 25 minutes. Let stand for 10 minutes before serving.

Make-Ahead Tip: Casserole can be assembled earlier in the day without the crumb topping, and refrigerated. To serve, sprinkle with topping, and bake as directed above, adding a few more minutes if you transfer the dish directly from the refrigerator to the oven.

Shepherd's Pie with Sweet Potato Topping

This is one of my favorites, and every time I serve it to friends, they say it's a keeper. The soy "meat" crumbles are the secret—lots of flavor without the saturated fat. There's only 1 gram of fat with 8 grams of fiber and less than 250 calories per serving. Certainly more prostate-healthy and heart-healthy than the original.

Serving Suggestions: For a crunchy accompaniment, try a green bean salad with chopped scallions, drizzled with a mustardy vinaigrette.

MAKES 8 SERVINGS
Prep: 15 minutes / Cook: 1 hour

Potato Topping:

1 pound sweet potatoes, peeled and cut into quarters

$\frac{1}{4}$ cup unsweetened soy milk

1 tablespoon light olive oil

$\frac{1}{2}$ teaspoon salt

Filling:

1 tablespoon light olive oil

1 sweet onion such as Vidalia, finely chopped

2 carrots, trimmed, peeled, and sliced

1 tablespoon tomato paste

$1\frac{1}{2}$ cups vegetable broth, homemade (page 101) or store-bought

$\frac{1}{2}$ teaspoon salt

$\frac{1}{4}$ teaspoon black pepper

1 tablespoon cornstarch

12 ounces ground soy "meat" crumbles

1 cup frozen green peas, thawed

1 cup frozen corn kernels, thawed

$\frac{1}{2}$ teaspoon dried rosemary

$\frac{1}{2}$ teaspoon dried thyme

Nonstick olive oil cooking spray

1. For the topping: Place potatoes in a saucepan and cover with cold water. Bring to a boil and cook until fork-tender, about 30 minutes. Drain and return to the saucepan. Mash with a potato masher, blending in soy milk, oil, and salt.

2. For the filling: Meanwhile, in a large skillet, heat oil over medium heat. Add onion and carrots and cook, stirring occasionally, until softened, about 5 minutes. Stir in tomato paste, broth, salt, and pepper.

3. In a small bowl, mix together cornstarch and 2 tablespoons of water and stir into the skillet. Simmer until slightly thickened, about 1 minute. Scrape into a large bowl. Stir in crumbles, peas, corn, rosemary, and thyme.

4. Heat oven to 375°F. Lightly coat a 13 x 9 x 2-inch baking dish with cooking spray. Spoon filling into the dish, spreading evenly. Spread mashed sweet potatoes over top.

5. Bake until bubbly and top is lightly colored, about 30 minutes. Let stand 5 minutes before serving.

Make-Ahead Tip: Pie can be assembled earlier in the day. If you take it directly from the refrigerator and put it in the oven, allow a little extra baking time.

Curried Vegetable Stew with Coconut

If you want to increase the protein in this dish, it's very easy to do—just cube 12 ounces of firm tofu and gently stir it into the vegetables in step 4 when they are tender, but before adding the coconut milk mixture. This recipe is based on one from my *Home Cooking Around the World: A Recipe Collection* (Stewart, Tabori & Chang, 2001).

Serving Suggestions: Spoon over brown basmati or jasmine rice and accompany with a spinach and tomato salad.

MAKES 6 SERVINGS

Prep: 20 minutes / Cook: about 25 minutes

1 boiling potato, peeled and cut into $\frac{1}{2}$-inch cubes

3 medium-size carrots, trimmed, peeled, and sliced $\frac{1}{4}$-inch thick

6 ounces green beans, trimmed and cut into $\frac{1}{2}$-inch pieces

1 sweet potato, peeled and cut into $\frac{1}{2}$-inch cubes

1 red bell pepper, cored, seeded, and cut into small squares

1 cup frozen peas

$\frac{1}{2}$ cup cold water

1 teaspoon ground turmeric (page 38)

1 teaspoon curry powder

1 teaspoon ground cumin

1–2 fresh hot green chile peppers such as serrano, cored, seeded, and finely chopped

$\frac{1}{4}$ cup canned regular or "lite" coconut milk

$\frac{1}{4}$ cup plain soy yogurt

1 teaspoon salt

1 small star fruit (carambola), thinly sliced or diced (optional)

1. In a large nonstick saucepan, combine white potato, carrots, beans, sweet potato, bell pepper, and peas.

2. In a 1-cup measure, combine the water, turmeric, and curry powder. Stir into vegetable mixture. Cover pan and bring to boiling. Lower heat and gently cook, covered, stirring occasionally, until vegetables are tender, 15 to 20 minutes.

3. Meanwhile, using a mortar and pestle or a small bowl and the back of a spoon, crush cumin and chiles together to form a paste. In a small bowl, stir together coconut milk, yogurt, and chile mixture.

4. When vegetables in the saucepan are tender, stir in coconut milk mixture and salt. Gently heat through, stirring occasionally.

5. Ladle into bowls and garnish with star fruit, if using.

Make-Ahead Tip: Stew can be refrigerated for up to a day. To serve, gently reheat in a saucepan, stirring occasionally, and do not let boil.

Edamame Moo Shu with Tortillas

Inspired by the classic Chinese stir-fry that mixes shredded pork, eggs, and a variety of other ingredients, this vegetarian version replaces the pork with edamame and nuts, creating a dish with 10 grams of fiber. Preparation is made even easier by using prepackaged broccoli slaw, and the slaw along with the cabbage makes for a significant serving of cruciferous vegetables and antioxidants. Instead of tortillas for the wrapper, you can use soft lettuce leaves, such as Boston lettuce. For added protein, stir in 8 ounces of cooked shrimp or scallops.

Serving Suggestions: For a quick, almost pickled salad, stir together thinly sliced radishes and cucumbers with rice vinegar.

MAKES 4 SERVINGS

Prep: 20 minutes / Cook: 12 minutes

> 2 tablespoons reduced-sodium soy sauce
>
> 2 teaspoons dry sherry or water
>
> 2 teaspoons peeled, grated fresh ginger
>
> 1 teaspoon honey
>
> 1 teaspoon cornstarch
>
> 2 teaspoons light olive oil
>
> 2 cups (4 ounces) sliced mushrooms, cleaned and tough stems removed
>
> 3 cups (7.5-ounce bag) broccoli slaw
>
> 2 cups thinly sliced green cabbage
>
> $1\frac{1}{2}$ cups frozen shelled and blanched edamame, thawed and blotted dry with paper towels
>
> 4 scallions, trimmed and thinly sliced
>
> $\frac{1}{3}$ cup chopped Brazil nuts or peanuts
>
> Bottled hoisin sauce, for serving
>
> Four 8-inch whole-wheat or white flour tortillas, warmed according to package directions

1. In a small dish, stir together soy sauce, sherry, ginger, honey, and cornstarch until cornstarch is dissolved. Set aside.

2. In a wok or large skillet, heat oil over medium-high heat. Add mushrooms and cook, stirring occasionally, until liquid from mushrooms is evaporated, about 4 minutes. Add

broccoli slaw and sliced cabbage and stir-fry for 3 minutes. Add edamame and scallions and stir-fry for 3 minutes more. Stir soy sauce mixture, add to wok, and cook, stirring, until thickened, about 1 minute. Stir in Brazil nuts. Remove from heat.

3. To serve, have each diner spread a spoonful of hoisin sauce down the center of each tortilla. Spoon about $\frac{3}{4}$ cup filling down the center. Fold sides over ends of filling and roll up, burrito-style.

Make-Ahead Tip: Filling can be made a day ahead and refrigerated. Gently reheat in a skillet to serve.

CHAPTER VII

FISH

FISH, WITH ITS SHORT COOKING TIME, is an easy fix, and there are abundant varieties to choose from now that most markets get an overnight delivery of fresh fish. Fish is essential to a prostate-healthy eating plan because it is a rich source of heart-healthy omega-3 essential fatty acids (page 33), which have significant antioxidant properties. The omega-3 content of a particular fish depends on how fatty it is. Generally, the darker the flesh, which usually means a fish from colder waters, the fattier it is, and that means a higher omega-3 concentration.

The American Heart Association and others generally recommend two or three servings of fish a week. However, there is some concern about the levels of PCBs and mercury in fish. Generally, larger fish are higher up the feeding chain and have higher levels of toxins—swordfish is an example. Also, there have been some reports that farm-raised salmon, as well as other farm-raised fish, have higher levels of PCBs than wild fish. Studies have found that the fishmeal fed to farmed salmon is often contaminated with PCBs. In addition, farm-raised fish are fattier than wild, and PCBs are stored in fat. There are a couple of things you can do about this. If you're sure you're eating farm-raised fish, remove the skin and trim all visible fat. Then, if you grill or broil fish, even more fat will drain away. And stock up on canned salmon, which more often than not is wild. All this should not scare you away from eating fish, because it is such a heart-healthy food, but rather help you to make it even more healthy.

As I've said, fish cooks quickly, making for less kitchen time—and it's easy to jazz up with lots of flavor, so even hesitant fish eaters will ask for seconds. Orange juice brings out the flavor, and I use it frequently as part of my cooking strategy, as in Haddock Fillets with Blood Oranges and Mustard (page 205). Lycopene-rich tomato partners well with fish, too: tasty examples are Roasted Monkfish with Tomatoes and Spices (page 210), and Cornmeal-Crusted Cod with Salsa (page 209). And for snacking, I always have on hand bottled pickled herring and canned sardines, which I arrange on crispy whole-grain flat breads, smeared with a mixture of soy mayonnaise, horseradish, and Dijon mustard.

If fish is not part of your eating plan already, then be sure to add it so you can benefit from its protein and omega-3s.

Baked Tuna with Honey Glaze and Moroccan Spices

The honey glaze mixture, with its touch of Moroccan spices, works best with a full-flavored fish—substitute salmon, mackerel, or bluefish for the tuna. And remember, darker-colored fish have a higher percentage of omega-3 fatty acids. There is just 1 gram of fat in this dish.

Serving Suggestions: Round out the plate with jasmine rice, as well as steamed snow peas tossed with cherry tomatoes and a little olive oil.

MAKES 4 SERVINGS

Prep: 5 minutes / Cook: 10 minutes

$\frac{1}{2}$ cup honey

$\frac{1}{2}$ teaspoon ground allspice

$\frac{1}{2}$ teaspoon ground cloves

$\frac{1}{4}$ teaspoon cayenne

1 pound tuna steaks

1. Heat oven to 425°F.

2. In a small bowl, stir together honey, 2 tablespoons water, allspice, cloves, and cayenne. Place fish in a baking dish just large enough to hold it in a single layer. Spread honey mixture over fish.

3. Bake until fish is opaque in the center and just begins to flake when prodded with a fork, about 10 minutes, depending on thickness of fish.

Baked Sea Bass with Tomato and Black Olives

This sauce contains lycopene from the tomatoes and "good" fat from the olives—monounsaturated. It also marries well with cod, haddock, halibut, monkfish, grouper, or tilapia. You can make the sauce on its own and toss it with whole-wheat pasta.

Serving Suggestions: Good choices for accompaniments include brown basmati rice or a chickpea and tomato salad, along with steamed fresh spinach.

MAKES 4 SERVINGS
Prep: 10 minutes / Cook: 40 minutes

> 1 teaspoon olive oil
>
> 1 medium-size onion, chopped
>
> 2 cloves garlic, finely chopped
>
> 1 can (about 15 ounces) crushed tomatoes in puree
>
> $\frac{3}{4}$ cup oil-cured black olives, pitted and chopped
>
> 1 tablespoon grated lemon zest
>
> $\frac{1}{4}$ teaspoon salt
>
> $\frac{1}{4}$ teaspoon black pepper
>
> $\frac{1}{2}$ cup packed basil leaves, or 1 tablespoon dried basil
>
> 1 pound sea bass fillets
>
> 2 tablespoons sliced almonds

1. In a medium-size nonstick saucepan, heat oil over medium heat. Add onion and cook, stirring occasionally, until softened, about 5 minutes. Add garlic and cook for 1 minute. Add tomatoes, olives, zest, salt, and pepper. Bring to a boil. Lower heat and simmer, uncovered, until thickened, about 20 minutes. Cut fresh basil into thin strips and stir into sauce or add the dried basil.

2. Heat oven to 425°F.

3. Place fish, skin side down, in a single layer in a baking dish. Spoon sauce over top.

4. Bake until fish is opaque in the center and begins to flake when prodded with fork, about 15 minutes, depending on thickness of fish.

5. Meanwhile, in a dry skillet, toast almonds over medium heat, stirring frequently, until lightly colored, about 3 minutes. Sprinkle over top of finished fish dish.

Make-Ahead Tip: The sauce can be made, without the addition of the fresh basil, up to two days ahead and refrigerated. To use, gently reheat, stirring in fresh basil.

Broiled Salmon with Cumin and Lemon

The combination of "sweet" spices accents the flavor of the salmon, which is an excellent source of omega-3 fatty acids. Search out wild salmon, which has higher levels of omega-3 and is less disease-prone than farm-raised. Tuna, mackerel, or tilapia can be substituted for the salmon. The dish qualifies as low-calorie, with only 150 calories.

Serving Suggestions: Accompany with corn kernels and chopped bottled roasted red pepper cooked together or corn on the cob, if in season, and thin sweet potato slices blanched and sauteed in a little light olive oil until slightly crisp.

MAKES 4 SERVINGS

Prep: 5 minutes / Refrigerate: 30 minutes / Cook: about 10 minutes

$\frac{1}{2}$ cup freshly squeezed lemon juice (2–3 lemons)

2 cloves garlic, finely chopped

1 teaspoon ground cumin

$\frac{1}{2}$ teaspoon ground coriander

$\frac{1}{4}$ teaspoon ground nutmeg

1 pound salmon fillets

1. In a glass baking dish just large enough to hold fish in a single layer, combine lemon juice, garlic, cumin, coriander, and nutmeg. Add fish, turning over to coat. Cover and refrigerate, turning occasionally, for 30 minutes.

2. Heat broiler.

3. Transfer fish, skin side down, to broiler-pan rack. Pour marinade into a small saucepan and boil for 2 minutes.

4. Meanwhile, broil fish about 4 inches from heat until it is opaque in the center and just begins to flake when prodded with a fork, 4 to 6 inches per side, depending on thickness of fish.

5. To serve, spoon boiled marinade over fish.

Jalapeño Salmon with Lime

The spicy jalapeño mixture is an easy way to perk up mildly flavored fish such as cod or halibut. Another 150-calorie dish.

Serving Suggestions: Either of these side dishes would provide color and cooling crunch: corn kernels with sautéed red bell pepper; or sliced jicama and cucumber drizzled with rice vinegar.

MAKES 4 SERVINGS

Prep: 5 minutes / Cook: about 10 minutes.

   2 tablespoons finely chopped, seeded fresh jalapeños or bottled pickled jalapeños
   1 tablespoon peeled, finely chopped fresh ginger
   2 cloves garlic, finely chopped
   1 teaspoon grated lime zest
   2 teaspoons freshly squeezed lime juice
   $\frac{1}{4}$ teaspoon salt
   1 pound salmon fillets or steak

1. Heat broiler or grill.

2. In a small bowl, combine jalapeño, ginger, garlic, lime zest and juice, and salt. Crush with the back of a spoon to form a paste. Rub over both sides of fish.

3. Broil or grill fish about 4 inches from heat until it is opaque in the center and begins to flake when prodded with a fork, 4 to 5 minutes per side, depending on thickness.

Jimmy's Baltimore Salmon Cakes

This recipe comes from a friend who grew up near Baltimore and knows about crab cakes—as he points out, this works for either crab or canned salmon. Since salmon is such a good source of omega-3s, it is called for here. You can remove the bones or mash them up in the salmon for a little extra calcium. Jimmy has two secrets in this recipe: the Old Bay Seasoning for flavor and the fat-free matzo meal for the crispy exterior. He also strongly suggests the yellow bell pepper for its color and its particular sweetness when cooked. In a pinch, you can substitute a red or orange bell pepper.

Serving Suggestions: Jimmy likes serving these cakes with coleslaw or potato salad (which for my purposes can be made with eggless soy-based mayonnaise), sugar snap peas, or succotash. Zucchini and Tomatoes with Sweet Potatoes and Herbs (page 240) would also be a good choice.

MAKES 8 CAKES

Prep: 20 minutes / Refrigerate: 30 minutes / Cook: about 5 minutes

1 can (about 15 ounces) salmon, drained, or 10–12 ounces lump crabmeat

2 tablespoons eggless soy-based mayonnaise

2 tablespoons bottled horseradish

1 tablespoon Dijon mustard

1 tablespoon hot red pepper sauce, or to taste

$\frac{1}{4}$ cup liquid egg substitute

Juice from $\frac{1}{2}$ lemon (about 2 tablespoons)

2 teaspoons Old Bay Seasoning

1 tablespoon baking powder

2 celery stalks, trimmed, peeled, and diced

1 yellow bell pepper, cored, seeded, and diced

$\frac{3}{4}$ to 1 cup whole-wheat bread crumbs (about 1 slice)

Matzo meal for coating

2 tablespoons light olive oil

1. In a medium-size bowl, mix together salmon, mayonnaise, horseradish, mustard, pepper sauce, egg substitute, and lemon juice, breaking up salmon. Mix in Old Bay Seasoning and baking powder. Mix in celery and bell pepper, then bread crumbs. You should have about 4 cups of mixture.

2. Shape mixture into eight $2\frac{1}{2}$-inch patties, using about $\frac{1}{2}$ cup mixture for each. Pat dry on paper towels. Spread matzo meal on a piece of waxed paper and coat patties with meal. Refrigerate for 30 minutes.

3. In a large nonstick skillet, heat oil over medium-high heat. Add patties, working in batches if necessary to avoid crowding skillet, and cook until heated through and lightly golden and crispy on both sides, 2 to 3 minutes per side. Serve immediately.

Make-Ahead Tip: Patties without the matzo meal coating can be made a day ahead and refrigerated. To cook, coat with meal and proceed as above.

Lemony Snapper with Vegetables in Packets

The fish remains moist and takes on some of the flavor of the vegetables and lemon because all the ingredients are steamed together in a sealed packet. And no messy cleanup. This recipe yields a main course along with a vegetable side dish for a total of 150 calories and only 3 grams of fat (1 gram saturated fat). Fish with delicate flesh, such as cod and sole, take well to steaming.

Serving Suggestions: Since the vegetables are already in the packet, all you need is some jasmine rice or whole-wheat couscous, or brown basmati rice.

MAKES 4 SERVINGS

Prep: 20 minutes / Cook: 30 minutes

> 2 medium-size carrots, trimmed, peeled, and cut into 2-inch-long, $\frac{1}{4}$-inch-square sticks
>
> 1 small red bell pepper, cored, seeded, and cut into thin strips
>
> 1 teaspoon light olive oil
>
> 1 teaspoon dried thyme
>
> $\frac{1}{2}$ teaspoon salt
>
> $\frac{1}{4}$ teaspoon black pepper
>
> 1 pound red snapper fillets
>
> $\frac{1}{4}$ cup vegetable broth, homemade (page 101) or store-bought, or dry vermouth
>
> 8 very thin lemon slices

1. Place a baking sheet in oven and heat oven to 400°F. Cut four 18 x 12-inch rectangles of heavy-duty aluminum foil.

2. In a medium-size bowl, toss together carrots, bell pepper, oil, thyme, salt, and pepper. Divide vegetables evenly among the pieces of foil, arranging them in the center. Divide fillets into four equal portions and place them, skin side down, over the top of the vegetables, trimming to fit, if necessary. Sprinkle with broth. Place 2 lemon slices on fish in each packet.

3. For each packet, bring two long sides of foil up and over fish, folding edges over together twice. Fold each short end over twice to form tightly sealed packets.

4. Place packets on the baking sheet in the oven and bake for 25 to 30 minutes. Carefully open one packet to check for doneness. Fish should be opaque in the center and just beginning to flake when prodded with a fork, and vegetables should be tender.

5. Carefully open each packet and place it on a dinner plate, and serve.

Make-Ahead Tip: Packets can be assembled 30 minutes before cooking. Refrigerate and allow a little extra time for baking the chilled packets.

Flounder with Fennel and Lemon

The marinade works with any fish, since fennel seems to be a perfect partner with things from the sea. One hundred and ten calories—that's all there is in this dish.

Serving Suggestions: To keep the menu light, steep couscous in hot vegetable broth with peas and serve alongside steamed asparagus or broccoli.

MAKES 4 SERVINGS
Prep: 5 minutes / Refrigerate: 30 minutes / Cook: about 10 minutes

> 1 tablespoon fennel seeds, crushed
>
> 2 teaspoons grated lemon zest
>
> 1 teaspoon dried thyme
>
> 1 teaspoon light olive oil
>
> $\frac{1}{2}$ teaspoon salt
>
> 1 pound flounder fillets
>
> Nonstick olive oil cooking spray

1. In a small bowl, combine fennel seeds, zest, thyme, oil, and salt. Rub mixture over fish, place in a glass dish, cover, and refrigerate for 30 minutes.
2. Heat broiler. Lightly coat the broiler-pan rack with nonstick cooking spray. Transfer fish, skin side down, to the rack.
3. Broil about 6 inches from heat until fish is opaque in the center and begins to flake when prodded with a fork, about 8 to 10 minutes, depending on thickness of fish.

Cod in Tomato-Ginger Sauce

The tomato makes this a lycopene-rich dish. The sauce is also delicious spooned over cooked vegetables or steamed or sauteed tofu. Halibut, haddock, or scrod can be substituted for the cod.

Serving Suggestions: Brown basmati rice, regular brown rice, or whole-wheat couscous, along with steamed carrots tossed with a little olive oil, Dijon mustard, and ground cumin are tasty additions to the menu.

MAKES 4 SERVINGS

Prep: 10 minutes / Cook: 25 minutes

2 teaspoons olive oil

1 large onion, finely chopped

2 cloves garlic, finely chopped

1 pound tomatoes, cored, seeded, and diced, or 1 can (14.5 ounces) diced tomatoes

$\frac{1}{4}$ cup orange juice

1 tablespoon soy sauce

1 tablespoon peeled, finely chopped fresh ginger

$\frac{1}{4}$ teaspoon salt

$\frac{1}{8}$ teaspoon black pepper

1 pound cod fillet

1. In a large nonstick skillet, heat oil over medium heat. Add onion and cook, stirring occasionally, until it is slightly softened, about 3 minutes. Add garlic and cook for 1 minute. Stir in tomatoes, orange juice, soy sauce, ginger, salt, and pepper. Bring to a boil. Lower heat and simmer, uncovered, stirring occasionally, for 10 minutes to blend flavors and slightly thicken.

2. Meanwhile, heat oven to 375°F.

3. Spoon $\frac{1}{2}$ cup sauce into a shallow baking dish or pie plate. Place fish, skin side down, over sauce, cutting to fit in dish, if necessary. Spoon remaining sauce over fish.

4. Bake until fish is opaque in the center and just begins to flake when prodded with a fork, 8 to 10 minutes, depending on thickness of fish.

Make-Ahead Tip: The sauce can be made up two days ahead and refrigerated. Gently reheat to use in recipe.

Halibut with Orange-Ginger Sauce

For this dish, the fish is poached or gently simmered in a flavored liquid. After the fish is cooked and removed, the cooking liquid is boiled to reduce and thicken it so it becomes a sauce. If you haven't tried this cooking method, add it to your repertoire, since it produces lots of flavor without fat. You can substitute cod, haddock, or grouper for the halibut.

Serving Suggestions: Couscous, brown basmati rice, or orzo would be good choices for soaking up the sauce, and for a vegetable side dish, sauteed green beans with garlic.

MAKES 4 SERVINGS
Prep: 10 minutes / Cook: 18 minutes

> 2 cups orange juice
> 1 tablespoon peeled, grated fresh ginger
> 1 tablespoon Dijon mustard
> $\frac{1}{4}$ teaspoon black pepper
> 1 pound halibut fillets

1. In a nonstick skillet just large enough to hold the fish in a single layer, stir together orange juice, ginger, mustard, and pepper. Bring to a boil. Add fish, skin side down, in a single layer and return to gentle boil. Lower heat, cover skillet, and gently simmer until fish is opaque in the center and flesh begins to flake when prodded with a fork, 6 to 10 minutes, depending on thickness of fish. Using a slotted spoon, remove fish to plate and cover with foil to keep warm. Cut into serving portions, if necessary.

2. Boil liquid over high heat until thickened to sauce consistency, about 8 minutes.

3. To serve, spoon sauce over fish.

Broiled Cod with Sun-Dried Tomato Sauce

Adding sun-dried tomatoes to the ordinary canned variety makes for an intensely flavored sauce with lots of lycopene. You can make the sauce on its own and toss with cooked whole-wheat pasta or even spread it on a sandwich for a topping. It also marries well with haddock, halibut, grouper, snapper, tilapia, or tuna.

Serving Suggestions: Steamed small new red potatoes tossed with chopped fresh parsley or fresh basil and your favorite green vegetable would complete the menu.

MAKES 4 SERVINGS (2 CUPS SAUCE)
Prep: 15 minutes / Cook: 40 minutes

Sauce:

1 teaspoon olive oil

1 onion, finely chopped

1 clove garlic, finely chopped

$\frac{1}{2}$ cup sun-dried tomatoes packed in oil, drained, blotted dry with paper towels, and chopped

1 can (about 15 ounces) whole tomatoes, in juice

$\frac{1}{2}$ teaspoon black pepper

1 tablespoon balsamic vinegar or red wine vinegar

Chopped fresh herbs, such as basil, mint, oregano, or flat-leaf parsley (optional)

Fish:

1 pound cod fillet

Nonstick olive oil cooking spray

1. For the sauce: In a medium-size skillet with a lid, heat oil over medium heat. Add onion and reduce heat. Cover skillet and cook, stirring occasionally, until onion is softened, about 5 minutes. Add garlic and cook, uncovered, for 30 seconds. And sun-dried tomatoes, canned tomatoes with their liquid, and pepper. Bring to a boil, breaking up tomatoes with a wooden spoon. Reduce heat and simmer, uncovered, until thickened, 20 to 25 minutes. Stir in vinegar and remove from heat. Stir in fresh herbs, if using, just before serving.

2. For the fish: Heat broiler. Coat the broiler-pan rack with cooking spray. Place cod, skin side down, on rack.

3. Broil fish about 4 inches from heat until it is opaque in the center and just begins to flake when prodded with a fork, 4 to 6 minutes per side, depending on thickness.

4. Serve fish with sauce.

Make-Ahead Tip: Sauce can be made up to three days ahead without vinegar or herbs, and refrigerated. Gently reheat in a saucepan, and then stir in vinegar and optional herb.

Scrod with Corn and Tomato

The tomato-corn sauce, full of lycopene, antioxidants, and fiber, is good spooned over any fish. In addition, it makes a good pasta topper, tossed with whole-wheat penne or rigatoni.

Serving Suggestions: For a side salad, toss together chickory and red leaf lettuce with a cider vinegar dressing.

MAKES 4 SERVINGS

Prep: 15 minutes / Refrigerate: 15 minutes / Cook: 20 minutes

1 tablespoon freshly squeezed lemon or lime juice

2 teaspoons light olive oil

$\frac{1}{2}$ teaspoon ground cumin

$\frac{1}{4}$ teaspoon ground cinnamon

$\frac{1}{4}$ teaspoon salt

1 pound scrod fillets

Nonstick olive oil cooking spray

Sauce:

1 tablespoon olive oil

$\frac{1}{2}$ pound zucchini, trimmed and cut into small dice

2 cups frozen corn kernels, thawed

1 can (14.5 ounces) Mexican-style stewed tomatoes

1. In a small bowl, stir together lemon juice, oil, cumin, cinnamon, and salt. Place fish on a baking sheet and brush with half the lemon mixture. Refrigerate for 15 minutes.

2. Heat broiler. Lightly coat the broiler-pan rack with cooking spray.

3. For the sauce: Meanwhile, in a medium-size nonstick skillet, heat oil over medium heat. Add zucchini and cook, stirring occasionally, until zucchini is slightly softened, about 3 minutes. Stir in corn and tomatoes. Bring to a boil. Lower heat and simmer vigorously until most of liquid boils off, about 5 minutes. Remove from heat and cover to keep warm.

4. Place fish, skin side down, on the broiler-pan rack. Broil fish about 4 inches from heat, basting occasionally with remaining lemon mixture, until fish is opaque in the center and begins to flake when prodded with a fork, 8 to 10 minutes, depending on thickness of fish.

5. To serve, spoon tomato mixture over fish.

Make-Ahead Tip: Tomato mixture can be refrigerated for up to two days.

Bluefish with Chipotle-Orange Sauce

You can substitute mackerel or haddock fillets for the bluefish. And keep in mind, this is not a dish for the faint-hearted when it comes to spicy heat—the canned chipotle chile used in the sauce is eye-watering. You can omit the chile and the dish will still be tasty.

Serving Suggestions: Since there is so much flavor in the dish, serve a strongly flavored vegetable, such as asparagus or broccoli, along with orzo seasoned with cumin or chili powder.

MAKES 4 SERVINGS
Prep: 10 minutes / Cook: about 15 minutes

> Nonstick olive oil cooking spray
> 1 tablespoon olive oil
> $\frac{1}{4}$ cup yellow cornmeal
> $\frac{1}{2}$ teaspoon salt
> 1 pound bluefish fillet, cut crosswise into 4 portions
> 1 canned chipotle chile in adobo sauce, chopped
> $\frac{1}{2}$ cup orange juice

1. Coat a large nonstick skillet with cooking spray. Add oil to skillet and heat over medium-high heat.

2. Meanwhile, on a sheet of waxed paper or large plate, stir together cornmeal and salt. Coat pieces of fish on both sides with mixture.

3. Add fish, skin side down, to the skillet, and cook, turning over once or twice, until fish is opaque in the center, just begins to flake when prodded with a fork, and cornmeal coating is lightly golden and crispy, 10 to 15 minutes, depending on thickness of fish. Transfer fish to a plate and loosely cover with foil to keep warm.

4. Add chile to the skillet and cook over medium heat, stirring, for 30 seconds. Add orange juice, scraping up any browned bits from the bottom of the skillet, and cook until liquid is reduced to a sauce with coating consistency, about 1 minute.

5. Place fish on serving plates and spoon sauce over top.

Broiled Tuna with Horseradish and Apple

The combination of apple and horseradish is usually paired with meats, especially pork, but it also teams up well with full-flavored fish. You can substitute mackerel or bluefish for the tuna, or even a more mild-flavored fish such as cod or halibut. Fish from deep, cold waters usually have a higher percentage of omega-3 fatty acids. Only three ingredients in this dish, and 138 calories and 1 gram of fat (no saturated fat)!

Serving Suggestions: Steamed broccoli tossed with a little lemon juice and brown basmati rice topped with chopped toasted Brazil nuts are easy-to-fix go-withs.

MAKES 4 SERVINGS

Prep: 5 minutes / Cook: about 10 minutes

> Nonstick olive oil cooking spray
>
> 1 pound tuna steaks, about 1 inch thick
>
> 1 tablespoon drained bottled horseradish, or more to taste
>
> 1 Granny Smith apple, peeled, cored, and grated

1. Heat broiler. Lightly coat the broiler-pan rack with cooking spray. Place fish on the rack.

2. In a small bowl, combine horseradish and apple. Spread half of mixture over one side of steaks.

3. Broil about 4 inches from heat for 4 minutes. Turn fish over and spread remaining horseradish mixture on top and broil until fish just begins to flake when prodded with a fork, 4 to 6 minutes, depending on thickness of fish.

Haddock Fillets with Blood Oranges and Mustard

This dish was invented when I was staying with friends in California and was asked if I would throw together a main course for a small dinner party that same day, in about four hours. We had about two hours to shop, and this is what I came up with when I spotted blood oranges in the market. Originally I used haddock, but when I returned home to the East Coast, I discovered that I also liked this dish with bluefish, which during the summer months where I live is caught almost daily. This recipe also works well with cod, mackerel, tuna, and mullet. If you live in Florida, you're fortunate to have access to mullet. It's a dark-fleshed fish with great flavor that especially benefits from a quick pan sauté. Blood oranges, usually imported from Spain, come into the markets for a brief time around January and February. Their flavor is tart-sweet, and the red-colored flesh adds a bright, colorful touch to any dish.

Serving Suggestions: Red rice or a baked sweet potato and lightly steamed green beans or broccoli couple well with the orange flavor in this fish dish.

MAKES 4 SERVINGS
Prep: 10 minutes / Cook: about 10 minutes

> Nonstick olive oil cooking spray
> 1 pound haddock fillets
> $\frac{1}{2}$ teaspoon salt
> $\frac{1}{2}$ cup orange juice
> $\frac{1}{4}$ cup Dijon mustard
> 3 blood oranges, small seedless oranges, or clementines, peeled, divided into
>   segments, and seeded, if necessary

1. Heat oven to 350°F. Line a baking pan with aluminum foil and lightly coat foil with cooking spray.

2. Season fillets on both sides with salt. Place fish, skin side down, on foil. Brush fillets with orange juice. Spread mustard over fish and arrange orange segments on top, piercing each segment with a fork so juice will ooze out during cooking.

3. Bake fish until it is opaque in the center and just begins to flake when prodded with a fork, 10 to 15 minutes, depending on thickness of fish.

Yogurt-Mustard Cod Fillets with Dill

The soy yogurt and lemon juice combine to create a pleasant sharpness that blends with the dill and mustard. With so much flavor, it's hard to believe this dish has less than 100 calories and contains only 1 gram of fat (no saturated fat). This recipe also works with flounder, halibut, and pollock.

Serving Suggestions: Pearl barley with finely chopped red bell pepper, and thinly sliced raw zucchini tossed with a lemony vinaigrette would both underscore the flavor of the fish.

MAKES 4 SERVINGS
Prep: 5 minutes / Cook: 8 minutes

> Nonstick olive oil cooking spray
>
> 1 pound cod fillets
>
> 3 tablespoons plain soy yogurt
>
> 2 tablespoons finely chopped scallions
>
> 1 tablespoon Dijon mustard
>
> 1 tablespoon finely chopped fresh dill, or 1 teaspoon dried
>
> 1 teaspoon freshly squeezed lemon juice
>
> $\frac{1}{4}$ teaspoon black pepper

1. Heat broiler. Lightly coat the broiler-pan rack with cooking spray. Arrange fillets, skin side down, in a single layer on the rack.

2. In a small bowl, stir together yogurt, scallions, mustard, dill, and lemon juice. Spread evenly over fillets. Sprinkle with pepper.

3. Broil fish about 4 inches from heat, without turning over, until fish is opaque in the center and begins to flake when prodded with a fork, 5 to 8 minutes, depending on thickness of fish.

Soy-Glazed Halibut with Shiitake Mushrooms

Honey and orange juice balance the edginess of the soy sauce, and nutritionally, the mushrooms add selenium.

Serving Suggestions: To continue the Asian theme, mix together broccoli sprouts, radish sprouts, or other sprouts, with thinly sliced radishes and season with rice vinegar. Round out the menu with cooked rice noodles tossed with a little dark sesame oil.

MAKES 4 SERVINGS
Prep: 10 minutes / Refrigerate: 30 minutes / Cook: 20 minutes

$\frac{1}{4}$ cup orange juice

2 tablespoons soy sauce

2 tablespoons honey

1 pound halibut steaks

2 teaspoons olive oil

$\frac{1}{4}$ pound shiitake or oyster mushrooms, trimmed, tough stems removed, and halved or quartered if large

2 cloves garlic, finely chopped

2 scallions, trimmed and thinly sliced, for garnish

1. In a medium-size bowl, combine orange juice, soy sauce, and honey. Add halibut and turn to coat. Refrigerate, covered, for 30 minutes. Transfer fish to a broiler-pan rack and reserve marinade.

2. Heat broiler. Broil fish about 4 inches from heat, without turning over, until browned on top, opaque in the center, and just beginning to flake when prodded with a fork, 4 to 6 minutes, depending on thickness of fish. Cut into four equal portions, if necessary. Remove to a serving platter, cover with foil, and keep warm.

3. Meanwhile, in a medium-size nonstick skillet, heat oil over medium-high heat. Add mushrooms and cook, stirring occasionally, until slightly softened, about 3 minutes. Add garlic and cook, stirring occasionally, until fragrant, about 1 more minute. Transfer mushrooms to the platter with fish.

4. Add reserved marinade to the skillet. Gently boil until marinade is syrupy, about 3 minutes. Pour over fish and mushrooms. Garnish with scallions.

Roasted Haddock with Spinach and Salsa

Once you've organized and prepped each of the three components in this dish, it goes together quickly just before serving. Make it for company or a special evening at home. Nutritional pluses lineup: lycopene and other antioxidants, as well as omega-3s.

Serving Suggestions: For an easy side dish, steep regular or whole-wheat couscous in boiling vegetable broth and then add some sauteed chopped scallions.

MAKES 4 SERVINGS

Prep: 20 minutes / Cook: 10 minutes

Fish:

Nonstick olive oil cooking spray

1 pound haddock, cod, scrod, or other mild-tasting white fish fillet

2 tablespoons olive oil

$\frac{1}{4}$ teaspoon salt

$\frac{1}{8}$ teaspoon black pepper

1 tablespoon Dijon mustard

Spinach:

1 tablespoon olive oil

2 cloves garlic, finely chopped

1 bag (12 ounces) fresh spinach, cleaned and tough stems removed

1 teaspoon ground cumin

$\frac{1}{2}$ teaspoon salt

$\frac{1}{4}$ teaspoon black pepper

2 teaspoons freshly squeezed lemon juice

Mexican Tomato Salsa with Serrano Chile (page 52)

1. For the fish: Heat oven to 400°F. Line a baking sheet with aluminum foil and lightly coat foil with cooking spray. Coat fish with olive oil and place, skin side down, on foil. Sprinkle with salt and pepper. Spread mustard over top.

2. Roast fish until it is opaque in the center and begins to flake when prodded with a fork, about 10 minutes, depending on thickness.

3. For the spinach: Meanwhile, heat oil in a large nonstick skillet over medium heat. Add garlic and cook, stirring frequently, for 1 minute, being careful not to let garlic burn. Add spinach, sprinkle with cumin, salt, and pepper, and cook, stirring frequently, until spinach wilts, 2 to 3 minutes. Remove from heat.

4. To serve, stir lemon juice into spinach. Spoon spinach onto a platter or four serving plates. Place fish on top and spoon salsa over fish. Serve immediately.

Cornmeal-Crusted Cod with Salsa

Supermarket shelves seem to be exploding with all new lines of bottled salsas. One of my favorite brands is the preservative-free Mrs. Renfro's, which is advertised as being made in Fort Worth, Texas since 1940. The selection includes roasted, habanero, and chipotle-corn, among others. Salsas are a great source of antioxidants, especially lycopene.

Serving Suggestions: Try an easy salad of blanched broccoli florets and cherry tomatoes tossed with Balsamic Vinaigrette (page 141), or Three Bean Salad with Edamame (page 129).

MAKES 4 SERVINGS
Prep: 10 minutes / Cook: about 15 minutes

$\frac{1}{4}$ cup liquid egg substitute

$\frac{1}{2}$ cup yellow cornmeal

2 teaspoons ground cumin

$\frac{1}{4}$ teaspoon salt

1 pound cod fillets or other firm-fleshed fish

2 tablespoons light olive oil

1 cup bottled salsa, heated if desired

1. Pour egg substitute into a medium-size bowl. Combine cornmeal, cumin, and salt on a plate or piece of waxed paper. Coat fish with egg substitute, then coat with cornmeal, and place on a clean piece of waxed paper.

2. In a medium-size nonstick skillet, heat oil. Add coated fillets and cook until coating is crispy and fish is opaque in the center and begins to flake when prodded with a fork, turning over as needed, about 15 minutes.

3. Cut fish into four serving portions and top with room temperature or heated salsa.

Roasted Monkfish with Tomatoes and Spices

Since monkfish is a firm-fleshed fish, it takes well to roasting at higher oven temperatures. The combination of spices is assertive, and you can vary the spicy heat by varying the amount of ground dried chile pepper. The tomato contributes lycopene, and drizzling the tomatoes with olive oil makes the lycopene more bioavailable. You can substitute cod, haddock, or sea bass for the monkfish.

Serving Suggestions: You need nothing much more than steamed broccoli, tossed with a little olive oil and chopped toasted almonds or with a splash of Ginger-Mustard Dressing (page 140).

MAKES 4 SERVINGS
Prep: 15 minutes / Cook: 25 minutes

> Nonstick olive oil cooking spray
> $\frac{1}{4}$ cup finely chopped fresh cilantro or parsley
> 3 cloves garlic, finely chopped
> 2 teaspoons ground cumin
> $\frac{1}{2}$ teaspoon ground coriander
> $\frac{1}{4}$ teaspoon ground dried chile pepper, or cayenne
> $\frac{1}{4}$ teaspoon ground cinnamon
> Pinch ground cloves, or allspice
> 1 pound monkfish fillet, rinsed and blotted dry with paper towels
> 1 large tomato, cored and coarsely chopped, or 1 can (14.5 ounces) diced tomatoes, drained
> 1 tablespoon olive oil
> 2 tablespoons freshly squeezed lemon juice
> $\frac{1}{4}$ teaspoon salt

1. Heat oven to 450°F. Line a baking pan with foil and coat with cooking spray.

2. Using a mortar and pestle or in a small bowl with the back of a metal spoon, crush together cilantro, garlic, cumin, coriander, chile pepper, cinnamon, and cloves. Rub spice mixture all over fish, and place fish, skin side down, on foil. Scatter tomato over fish, drizzle with oil and lemon juice, and sprinkle with salt.

3. Roast until fish is opaque in the center and just begins to flake when prodded with a fork, about 25 minutes.

Steamed Fish in Lettuce Wraps with Thai-Style Dipping Sauce

This is an extremely versatile dish that's fun for entertaining. Firm-fleshed fish such as tuna and monkfish hold together better in the lettuce wraps than flakier fish such as cod or flounder, but almost any fillet of fish or boneless fish steak can be used. Try sea bass, grouper, tilapia, orange roughy, turbot, or even shrimp. Shredded carrot or daikon radish, thinly sliced scallions or raw snow peas, and fresh basil and mint leaves are just some of the vegetables and herbs that can be added to the platter and wrapped with the fish in addition to cucumber, red or yellow bell pepper, and fresh cilantro.

Serving Suggestions: All you need to serve on the side is a bowl of rice—jasmine, brown basmati, white, or brown—a spoonful of which can also be added to the wrap.

MAKES 4 SERVINGS

Prep: 20 minutes / Cook: 15 minutes

> $1\frac{1}{2}$ pounds thick fish fillets or boneless fish steaks such as tuna, monkfish, sea bass, or tilapia
>
> 1 scallion, trimmed and finely chopped
>
> 1 tablespoon peeled, finely chopped fresh ginger
>
> 1 tablespoon soy sauce
>
> 1 head soft lettuce such as green leaf, red leaf, or Boston, separated into leaves
>
> 2 cups fresh cilantro sprigs
>
> 1 red bell pepper, cored, seeded, and cut into thin 2-inch strips
>
> 1 cucumber, peeled, halved lengthwise, seeded, and cut into thin 2-inch-long strips
>
> Thai-Style Dipping Sauce with Cilantro (page 51)

1. Arrange fish, skin side down if using fillets, on a steamer rack. Sprinkle with scallion, ginger, and soy sauce. Cover and steam until fish is opaque in the center and begins to flake when prodded with a fork, 5 to 10 minutes or longer, depending on thickness of fish.

2. Meanwhile, arrange lettuce leaves, cilantro, bell pepper, and cucumber on one side of serving platter. Transfer fish to the platter. Cut it into smaller pieces.

3. Allow each diner to wrap her or his own fish, cilantro, and vegetables in lettuce leaves. Be careful not to overstuff the leaves. Dip wraps into the sauce and eat with your hands.

PASTA & PIZZA

PASTA IS MORE THAN JUST SPAGHETTI, and that's what this chapter is about. But first, one caveat. Regardless of the trendy emphasis these days on low-carbohydrate diets and the million-dollar industry that has sprung up around them, keep in mind that pasta is a good source of protein, fiber, and complex carbohydrate. And it's low-fat, as long as you pay attention to what you spoon over the pasta. Portion control is often where people get in trouble. A single serving is not 8 ounces—make it 2 to 3 ounces of uncooked pasta, and you're on the right track.

Pasta is now available in whole-wheat versions in a variety of shapes with more nutrients and fiber per serving—5 to 7 grams of fiber as opposed to the usual 2 grams in refined pasta. Whole-wheat pasta retains the entire grain seed or kernel—usually eliminated when the pasta is refined—which includes the bran and the germ, where a whole host of vitamins, minerals, and fiber reside.

You can keep preparation easy by using a bottled pesto sauce or a meatless marinara sauce. Just be sure to check the label so you know what you're getting in terms of calories. Putting together quick sauces with your own flavor combinations can be almost as easy as opening a jar. Examples of quick are Penne with Mushrooms and Gremolata (page 214), and Penne with Red Bell Pepper Sauce and Brazil Nuts (page 221). For other pasta sauces, try the tomato and black olives (page 191), corn and tomato (page 202), and sun-dried tomato (page 200) sauces in Chapter VII.

For the baked party pastas, there are Mushroom Lasagna with Red Bell Pepper and Edamame (page 222) and Spinach and Mushroom Manicotti (page 224), which substitutes tofu for the cheese.

Anytime you want to sprinkle your pasta with grated Parmesan, reach for the grated Parmesan-style soy cheese—it's a good substitute. My favorite brand is Galaxy Nutritional Foods. But it does contain casein, which is a milk solid. So, if you're on a dairy-free diet, look for a vegan alternative. Another easy add-in for soy protein is a sprinkle of shelled edamame, fresh or thawed frozen.

The chapter concludes with a selection of pizzas made with a no-rise homemade whole-wheat crust and lycopene-rich tomatoes. Using soy cheese alternatives lets you still indulge in a Sunday night pizza party without all the usual saturated fat.

Just a final note: Some of the recipes in this chapter may register slightly high in grams of fat, but the fat is heart-healthy monounsaturated and polyunsaturated, rather than saturated.

Penne with Mushrooms and Gremolata

Gremolata is a mixture of chopped garlic, lemon zest, and parsley that adds a fresh accent to any dish. Garlic is a member of the lily family and contains the phytochemical allicin, thought by some to reduce the risk of cancer. And this pasta dish doesn't stop there: Mushrooms are a good source of selenium, and there are 8 grams of fiber per serving.

Serving Suggestion: Toss together a salad of bottled roasted red peppers, marinated artichoke hearts, and olives, and accompany with thin, crispy breadsticks.

MAKES 4 SERVINGS
Prep: 15 minutes / Cook: 12 minutes

8 ounces whole-wheat penne, linguine, or other pasta

1 tablespoon olive oil

4 scallions, trimmed and finely chopped

$\frac{1}{4}$ pound cremini, portobello mushrooms, or white button mushrooms, cleaned, tough stems removed, and mushrooms sliced

$\frac{1}{2}$ teaspoon salt

$\frac{1}{4}$ teaspoon black pepper

Gremolata (page 265)

1. In a large pot of lightly salted boiling water, cook pasta according to package directions.

2. Meanwhile, in a large nonstick skillet, heat oil over medium–high heat. Add scallions and cook, stirring occasionally, until softened, about 3 minutes. Add mushrooms and cook, stirring occasionally, until softened, about 3 minutes. Stir in salt and pepper.

3. Drain pasta, reserving $\frac{1}{4}$ cup cooking liquid. Add pasta, reserved liquid, and Gremolata to mushrooms in skillet, and toss to combine. Serve immediately.

Spaghetti with Herbed and Parmesan "Meatballs"

Here's a family favorite, but with special "meatballs." This recipe can be easily stretched to six servings—just increase the amount of pasta to 12 ounces.

Serving Suggestions: Crusty bread and a green salad—the usual.

MAKES 4 SERVINGS
Prep: 25 minutes / Cook: 15 minutes

8 ounces whole-wheat spaghetti, fettuccine, or other pasta

Herbed and Parmesan "Meatballs" in Tomato Sauce (page 178)

Grated Parmesan-style soy cheese, for sprinkling

1. Bring a large pot of lightly salted water to boiling and cook pasta according to package directions. Drain well and return to pot. Add a little tomato sauce and toss to coat pasta.
2. Spoon into pasta bowls or onto large plates and top with remaining sauce and meatballs. Pass the cheese.

Rigatoni with Broccoli and Sun-Dried Tomato–Black Olive Sauce

Turn to page 44 for the olive-sun-dried tomato spread recipe, or look in the Italian section of your supermarket for a bottled black olive spread, preferably with sun-dried tomatoes so you get a hit of lycopene. The olives are "fatty," but it's the beneficial monounsaturated variety. And of course, broccoli, a cruciferous vegetable, offers its usual array of antioxidants and other beneficial phytonutrients. This pasta combination is on the plates in the time it takes to cook the pasta. And remember, part of calorie-control is portion control—2 ounces uncooked pasta is sufficient for each serving.

Serving Suggestions: Whole-grain breadsticks and a combination of torn escarole and romaine with a sprinkling of shredded fresh basil leaves, drizzled with vinegar and oil, completes a meal that any trattoria would be proud to serve.

MAKES 4 SERVINGS

Prep: 10 minutes / Cook: 12 minutes

- 2 tablespoons olive oil
- 2 cloves garlic, finely chopped
- 2 small heads broccoli, tops cut into small florets and stems trimmed, peeled, and cut into thin coins
- $\frac{1}{4}$ cup vegetable broth, homemade (page 101) or store-bought
- 8 ounces whole-wheat rigatoni, penne, spaghetti, or other whole-grain pasta
- $\frac{3}{4}$ cup Black-Olive Spread with Sun-Dried Tomatoes (page 44), or bottled black olive spread (preferably with sun-dried tomatoes)
- $\frac{1}{4}$ cup grated Parmesan-style soy cheese, plus extra for garnish
- $\frac{1}{4}$ teaspoon black pepper

1. In a large skillet, heat oil over medium heat. Add garlic and cook, stirring, for 1 minute. Add broccoli and broth and stir to mix. Cover skillet and cook, stirring occasionally, until broccoli is fork-tender, about 5 minutes.

2. Meanwhile, in a large pot of lightly salted boiling water, cook pasta according to package directions. Drain, reserving $\frac{1}{2}$ cup cooking liquid.

3. Return pasta to the cooking pot. Add broccoli mixture, black olive spread, and $\frac{1}{4}$ cup cheese, stirring gently to mix. If pasta mixture is too dry, add a little of the reserved cooking liquid.

4. Spoon into serving bowls and sprinkle with black pepper and additional Parmesan cheese.

Rotelle with Sausage and Red Bell Pepper

The bell peppers are an excellent source of vitamin C and other antioxidants. Meatless soy sausage is tasty and without all the saturated fat.

Serving Suggestions: In a large salad bowl, toss together a variety of greens, or try one of the prepackaged organic greens combos, drizzled with a little vinegar and oil and topped with toasted sliced almonds or toasted chopped Brazil nuts.

MAKES 8 SERVINGS
Prep: 10 minutes / Cook: 15 minutes

1 tablespoon olive oil

2 medium-size onions, thinly sliced

3 large red bell peppers, cored, seeded, and thinly sliced, or a mixture of different-colored peppers

2 cloves garlic, finely chopped

1 teaspoon dried basil, crumbled

$\frac{1}{2}$ pound Italian-style soy sausage links, sliced

$\frac{1}{2}$ cup pitted black olives, coarsely chopped

1 tablespoon balsamic vinegar

$\frac{1}{4}$ teaspoon salt

$\frac{1}{4}$ teaspoon black pepper

1 pound whole-wheat rotelle or farfalle

Grated Parmesan-style soy cheese, for serving

1. In a large nonstick skillet, heat oil over medium–high heat. Add onions and cook, stirring frequently, until softened and lightly golden, about 5 minutes. Add bell peppers, garlic, and basil, and cook, stirring occasionally, for 5 minutes. Add sausage and cook, stirring, until peppers are very tender, about 10 minutes. Remove the skillet from heat. Stir in olives, vinegar, salt, and pepper.

2. Meanwhile, in a large pot of lightly salted boiling water, cook pasta according to package directions. Drain, reserving $\frac{1}{4}$ cup cooking water.

3. Return pasta to the pot, along with the reserved cooking water and sausage mixture, and toss to combine. Serve with grated Parmesan cheese on the side.

Make-Ahead Tip: Pepper and sausage sauce can be prepared a day ahead and refrigerated. Gently reheat in a saucepan, adding a little water if mixture seems too dry.

Rigatoni with Spinach and Lima Beans

Lima beans—the meaty, underutilized bean that is chock-full of protein, fiber, and minerals. And the frozen version is very convenient—purchase the big plastic bags so you always have them on hand in your freezer. Thawed, they make a great salad add-in.

Serving Suggestions: A pleasantly bitter combination of radicchio—the purple lettuce that comes in small, compact heads—and arugula is a nice counterpoint to the rich-tasting limas.

MAKES 4 SERVINGS
Prep: 10 minutes / Cook: 12 minutes

> 8 ounces whole-wheat rigatoni or penne
> $1/2$ recipe Sauteed Lima Beans and Spinach with Red Bell Pepper (page 239)
> $1/4$ cup vegetable broth, homemade (page 101), store-bought, or water
> Grated Parmesan-style soy cheese

1. In a large pot of lightly salted boiling water, cook pasta according to package directions.
2. Meanwhile, in a large nonstick skillet, gently reheat lima bean mixture with broth or water.
3. Drain pasta, reserving $1/2$ cup cooking water. Return pasta to the pot. Stir in lima bean mixture, and if the dish seems a little dry, stir in a little of the cooking water.
4. Spoon into serving bowls or onto plates and pass the cheese.

Penne with Carrot and White Bean Sauce

A hearty pasta dish, aromatically seasoned with dried sage. If you're growing little pots of fresh, by all means use that instead of the dried. The cannellini beans help to boost the fiber to 9 grams per serving.

Serving Suggestions: For a little zip in this menu, toss cherry or pear tomatoes with grated lemon zest and a drizzle of extra-virgin olive oil for a side salad.

MAKES 4 SERVINGS
Prep: 10 minutes / Cook: 20 minutes

2 tablespoons olive oil

1 onion, finely chopped

2 cloves garlic, finely chopped

2 carrots, trimmed, peeled, halved lengthwise, and thinly sliced crosswise

8 ounces whole-wheat penne, rigatoni, spaghetti, or other whole-grain pasta

1 can (16 ounces) cannellini beans, drained and rinsed

1 cup vegetable broth, homemade (page 101) or store-bought

$\frac{3}{4}$ teaspoon dried sage

$\frac{1}{4}$ teaspoon salt

2 tablespoons freshly squeezed lemon juice (1 lemon)

$\frac{1}{2}$ cup grated Parmesan-style soy cheese

3 tablespoons chopped fresh parsley

1. In a large nonstick skillet, heat oil over medium heat. Add onion and cook, stirring occasionally, until softened, about 5 minutes. Add garlic and cook, stirring frequently, for 1 minute. Add carrots and cook, stirring occasionally, for 5 minutes.

2. Meanwhile, in a large pot of lightly salted boiling water, cook pasta according to package directions.

3. To carrot mixture in the skillet, add beans, broth, sage, and salt, mashing about a quarter of the beans with a wooden spoon to thicken sauce. Cook, stirring occasionally, for 5 minutes. Stir in lemon juice and cook for 1 minute. Stir in cheese and parsley.

4. Drain pasta and return it to the pot. Add bean mixture, toss to combine, and serve.

Rotelle with Broccoli and Sun-Dried Tomato Pesto

Quick pasta dishes for that what-can-I-fix-tonight moment when you walk through the door at the end of the day, are made even quicker by using some of the bottled convenience sauces from supermarket shelves. Just make sure to have a supply of them in your cupboard or pantry. This dish is a good example, and the mix of broccoli with sun-dried tomatoes and whole-wheat pasta adds lots of health value, including a whopping 13 grams of fiber per serving.

Serving Suggestions: For a salad accompaniment, toss together Boston lettuce with red leaf lettuce, add your favorite low-fat dressing, and garnish with toasted chopped Brazil nuts.

MAKES 4 SERVINGS
Prep: 10 minutes / Cook: 12 minutes

> 8 ounces whole-wheat rotelle, rigatoni, or penne
> 1 pound broccoli, cut into small florets and stems trimmed, peeled, and cut into thin coins
> 1 cup bottled sun-dried tomato pesto
> $\frac{1}{4}$ teaspoon black pepper
> Grated Parmesan-style soy cheese, for garnish (optional)

1. In a large pot of lightly salted boiling water, cook pasta according to package directions. About 4 minutes before the end of the cooking time, add broccoli and continue cooking. Drain, reserving $\frac{1}{4}$ cup cooking water.

2. Return pasta and broccoli to the pot. Stir in pesto. For a thinner sauce, stir in a little of the cooking water. Add pepper and spoon into serving bowls. Pass the cheese, if using.

Penne with Red Bell Pepper Sauce and Brazil Nuts

The sauce, rich in lycopene, vitamin C, and other antioxidants, is ready by the time the pasta cooks. The Brazil nuts are a great source of selenium.

Serving Suggestions: A spinach salad with tomato and red onion rings makes a colorful accompaniment. Serve the pasta chilled or at room temperature and it becomes a pasta salad.

MAKES 4 SERVINGS
Prep: 10 minutes / Cook: 12 minutes

8 ounces whole-wheat penne, rigatoni, spaghetti, or other whole-grain pasta

2 tablespoons olive oil

2 cloves garlic, crushed

$\frac{1}{3}$ cup Brazil nuts, coarsely chopped

1 jar (12 ounces) roasted red peppers, drained and blotted dry

$\frac{1}{2}$ cup vegetable broth, homemade (page 101) or store-bought

3 tablespoons tomato paste

1 tablespoon balsamic vinegar

$\frac{1}{2}$ teaspoon salt

1. In a large pot of lightly salted boiling water, cook pasta according to package directions.
2. Meanwhile, in a large nonstick skillet, heat oil over medium heat. Add garlic and cook, stirring frequently, until lightly golden, 2 to 3 minutes. Add nuts and cook until lightly colored, about 2 minutes.
3. Transfer mixture to a food processor. Add red peppers, broth, tomato paste, vinegar, and salt. Puree and then scrape into a large serving bowl.
4. Drain pasta well. Add to sauce and toss to combine. Serve hot, warm, or even at room temperature.

Make-Ahead Tip: Sauce can be refrigerated for up to three days. To serve, gently reheat in a large saucepan, then toss with pasta.

Mushroom Lasagna with Red Bell Pepper and Edamame

No-boil lasagna noodles cut back on the usual lasagna-making time—no need to precook the noodles. And this dish, excellent for a family gathering or company, has almost none of the usual saturated fat (only 1 gram per serving): soy milk and soy cheese do the trick. Edamame (page 30) add a touch of green as well as protein and isoflavones, with their suspected cancer-fighting qualities. The mushrooms add selenium, and once you've tried the recipe, make it again with a variety of other mushrooms that are now available in supermarkets, such as cremini, shiitake, oyster, and the usual white button. Leftovers are delicious reheated in a microwave or 350°F oven.

Serving Suggestions: Toss a salad of radicchio, endive, and arugula with Balsamic Vinaigrette (page 141), or for faster prep, use a prepackaged salad mix that includes radicchio. For a milder-flavored salad, select a variety of dark, leafy greens such as Boston, Bibb, or red leaf and add halved cherry tomatoes.

MAKES 8 SERVINGS

Prep: 20 minutes / Cook: 65 minutes / Stand: 30 minutes

1 tablespoon olive oil

1 large red bell pepper, cored, seeded, and thinly sliced into 2-inch-long strips

1 large sweet onion such as Vidalia, quartered and thinly sliced

2 cloves garlic, finely chopped

1 cup frozen shelled and blanched edamame

$\frac{1}{2}$ teaspoon salt

$1\frac{3}{4}$ cups unsweetened soy milk

3 tablespoons all-purpose flour

$\frac{1}{2}$ teaspoon dried thyme

$\frac{1}{2}$ teaspoon dried rosemary, crushed

$\frac{1}{2}$ cup plus 2 tablespoons grated Parmesan-style soy cheese

Nonstick olive oil cooking spray

1 jar (about 26 ounces) meatless tomato marinara sauce, or 1 recipe Homemade All-Purpose Tomato Sauce (page 259)

2 tablespoons water

6 no-boil lasagna noodles (7 x $3\frac{1}{2}$-inches)

$1\frac{1}{2}$ cups (about 6 ounces) shredded mozzarella-syle soy cheese

2 portobello mushrooms, cleaned, tough stems removed, and thinly sliced

1. In a large nonstick skillet, heat oil over medium heat. Add bell pepper, onion, and garlic and cook, stirring occasionally, until slightly softened, about 5 minutes. Stir in edamame and salt and cook, stirring occasionally, until vegetables are just tender, about another 5 minutes. Transfer to a bowl and set aside.

2. Shake together $\frac{1}{2}$ cup of the soy milk and flour in a jar or container with tight-fitting lid until well blended with no lumps. Pour into the same skillet (no need to clean it), along with the remaining soy milk, the thyme, and rosemary. Set over medium heat and bring to a simmer, stirring constantly, then continue to gently simmer, stirring frequently, until thickened, about 2 minutes. Remove from heat. Stir in the $\frac{1}{2}$ cup Parmesan until well blended and smooth.

3. Heat oven to 375°F. Coat an 8 x 8 x 2-inch-square baking dish with cooking spray.

4. In the prepared dish, stir together $\frac{1}{2}$ cup of the tomato sauce and the 2 tablespoons water. Place two lasagna noodles, side by side, in the dish. Spoon half of the red pepper mixture over noodles and spread in an even layer. Drizzle with half of the Parmesan white sauce. Sprinkle with $\frac{1}{2}$ cup of the mozzarella. Arrange half of the portobello slices on top. Spoon on another $\frac{1}{2}$ cup tomato sauce and spread evenly. Repeat with two noodles, remaining red pepper mixture, remaining white sauce, $\frac{1}{2}$ cup mozzarella, remaining portobello slices, and $\frac{1}{2}$ cup tomato sauce. Top with the remaining two lasagna noodles. Spoon on the remaining cup tomato sauce and spread evenly. Cover dish tightly with foil.

5. Bake until hot in the center (an instant-read thermometer inserted in the center should register 180°F), about 55 minutes. Remove foil and sprinkle the top of the lasagna with the remaining $\frac{1}{2}$ cup mozzarella and 2 tablespoons Parmesan. Lightly coat a clean sheet of foil with cooking spray and place it, coated side down, over lasagna. Let stand until lasagna becomes firm, 20 to 30 minutes, then serve.

Make-Ahead Tip: Lasagna can be assembled through step 4 up to a day ahead and refrigerated. Let it come to room temperature before baking, or if you transfer it directly from the refrigerator to the oven, allow as much as 30 minutes extra baking time.

Spinach and Mushroom Manicotti

In this dish, which is great for entertaining, the tofu in the filling mimics the texture of the usual cheese. The tomato sauce provides lycopene; the spinach, phytonutrients; and the mushrooms, selenium.

Serving Suggestions: Toss together a huge green salad with tomatoes and Balsamic Vinaigrette (page 141), or a vegetable salad with broccoli, red bell pepper, carrots, and cherry tomatoes.

MAKES 8 SERVINGS
Prep: 20 minutes / Cook: about 40 minutes

- 1 box (8 ounces) manicotti pasta tubes (about 14), or 24 jumbo pasta shells
- 4 teaspoons olive oil
- 1 large onion, finely chopped
- 1 teaspoon salt
- 3 cloves garlic, finely chopped
- 2 boxes (10 ounces each) frozen chopped spinach, or 3 cups frozen chopped spinach from 16-ounce bag, thawed and squeezed dry
- 14 ounces firm tofu, drained, blotted dry with paper towels, and cut into cubes
- 2 large egg whites
- 1 tablespoon dried oregano, crumbled
- $\frac{1}{4}$ teaspoon black pepper
- $\frac{1}{8}$ teaspoon ground nutmeg
- $\frac{1}{2}$ pound portobello or other mushrooms, cleaned, tough stems removed, and mushrooms coarsely chopped
- Homemade All-Purpose Tomato Sauce (page 259), or 1 jar (26 ounces) meatless tomato marinara sauce
- Grated Parmesan-style soy cheese, for serving (optional)

1. In a large pot of lightly salted boiling water, cook manicotti or shells according to package directions. Drain in a colander and rinse under cold running water to stop cooking.
2. Meanwhile, in a large nonstick skillet, heat 2 teaspoons of the oil over medium-high heat. Add onion and salt and cook, stirring occasionally, until softened, about 5 minutes. Add garlic and cook, stirring, for 1 minute. Add spinach and cook, stirring to break up clumps, for 2 minutes. Transfer mixture to a food processor. Wipe out skillet.

3. Add tofu, egg whites, oregano, pepper, and nutmeg to the food processor. Pulse until pureed. Scrape mixture into a large bowl.

4. In the skillet, heat the remaining 2 teaspoons oil over medium-high heat. Add mushrooms and cook, stirring occasionally, until softened and browned, about 5 minutes. Fold mushrooms into spinach mixture until evenly distributed. You should have about 4 cups filling.

5. Heat oven to 350°F. Spoon a little tomato sauce over the bottom of 13 x 9 x 2-inch baking dish. Stuff each manicotti with $\frac{1}{3}$ cup filling, spooning filling in from either end, and place in the baking dish. (Or fill each shell with about $2\frac{1}{2}$ tablespoons.) Spoon remaining tomato sauce over manicotti. Cover the dish with aluminum foil.

6. Bake until heated through and sauce is bubbling around the edges, about 30 minutes. Let stand for 10 minutes before serving. Sprinkle with Parmesan, if desired.

Make-Ahead Tip: Manicotti tubes and filling can be prepared separately a day ahead, or the whole dish can be assembled earlier in the day and refrigerated. Let it come to room temperature before baking, or add a little extra baking time if you put the dish in the oven directly from the refrigerator.

Roasted Red Pepper Pizza

The roasted red peppers and tomato sauce provide a lineup of antioxidants, as well as good flavor.

Serving Suggestions: Toss together pieces of romaine lettuce, pitted black olives, halved cherry tomatoes, and a vinaigrette for an easy salad.

MAKES 8 SLICES

Prep: 15 minutes / Cook: about 15 minutes

Yellow cornmeal, for pizza pan

$\frac{1}{2}$ recipe Whole-Wheat Pizza Dough (page 229), or one 12-inch store-bought prepared pizza crust

$\frac{1}{2}$ cup (2 ounces) shredded mozzarella-style soy cheese

$\frac{1}{2}$ cup (2 ounces) shredded Swiss- or provolone-style soy cheese

1 tablespoon grated Parmesan-style soy cheese

$\frac{1}{2}$ cup Homemade All-Purpose Homemade Tomato Sauce (page 259), or bottled meatless pizza sauce

1 jar (7 ounces) roasted red peppers, drained and blotted dry with paper towels

$\frac{1}{2}$ small red onion, thinly sliced and separated into rings

1. Heat oven to 500°F. Place oven rack in lowest position.

2. Sprinkle a little cornmeal on a 12-inch pizza pan. Pat out dough evenly in pan, forming an edge all around.

3. Bake dough until lightly browned and crisp, about 5 minutes.

4. In a small bowl, combine cheeses.

5. Spread tomato sauce over crust, leaving a $\frac{1}{2}$-inch border all around. Sprinkle with cheeses. Arrange peppers on top and sprinkle with onion.

6. Return to oven and bake until topping is heated through and edge of crust is browned, 10 to 12 minutes. Let stand for 5 minutes before cutting.

Broccoli Rabe Pizza with Tomato

Broccoli rabe has a slightly bitter taste that marries well with all the cheeses in this pizza—it's also a great source of phytonutrients. If you like, you can substitute a pound (4 to 5 cups) of broccoli florets or broccolini for the broccoli rabe.

Serving Suggestions: A big spinach salad with sliced red onion and sliced white button or cremini mushrooms is a great addition on the side.

MAKES 8 SLICES
Prep: 15 minutes / Cook: about 15 minutes

> Yellow cornmeal, for pizza pan
> $\frac{1}{2}$ recipe Whole-Wheat Pizza Dough (page 229), or one 12-inch store-bought crust
> $1\frac{1}{2}$ pounds broccoli rabe, thick stems removed
> 1 teaspoon olive oil
> 3 cloves garlic, sliced
> $\frac{1}{4}$ teaspoon salt
> $\frac{1}{8}$ teaspoon black pepper
> $\frac{1}{2}$ cup (about 2 ounces) shredded Swiss-style soy cheese
> $\frac{1}{2}$ cup (about 2 ounces) shredded mozzarella-style soy cheese
> $\frac{1}{3}$ cup grated Parmesan-style soy cheese
> 2 medium-size tomatoes, cored, halved, and thinly sliced, or $\frac{1}{2}$ pound cherry
>   tomatoes, sliced

1. Heat oven to 500°F. Place oven rack in lowest position.

2. Sprinkle a 12-inch pizza pan with a little cornmeal. Pat out dough evenly into pan, creating a slight edge all around.

3. Bake dough until lightly browned and crisp, about 5 minutes.

4. Meanwhile, in a large pot of boiling water, blanch broccoli rabe until crisp-tender, 3 minutes. Drain well. Coarsely chop.

5. In a large nonstick skillet, heat oil over medium heat. Add garlic and cook, stirring frequently, for 1 minute. Add broccoli rabe, salt, and pepper and cook, stirring, for 2 minutes.

6. In a small bowl, combine cheeses. Sprinkle half over crust, leaving $\frac{1}{2}$-inch border all around. Top with broccoli rabe. Arrange tomatoes on top and sprinkle with remaining cheese.

7. Return to oven and bake until cheese is melted, topping is heated through, and edge of crust is browned, 8 to 10 minutes. Let stand 5 minutes before cutting.

Tomato Skillet Pizza with Mozzarella and Basil

The tomato in this pizza is a great vehicle for the antioxidant lycopene, thought by some experts to have prostate cancer–fighting properties. The recipe calls for a 9-inch cast-iron skillet, but the pizza can be prepared in a regular 12-inch pizza pan. If you grow your own tomatoes, this is the place to use them. You can also substitute yellow or orange cherry or pear tomatoes if they are available.

Serving Suggestions: Reach for one of the prepackaged organic salad mixes in the produce department, toss with your favorite salad dressing (preferably low-fat), and there you have your pizza accompaniment.

MAKES 8 SLICES

Prep: 15 minutes / Cook: about 15 minutes

> Yellow cornmeal, for skillet
>
> $1/2$ recipe Whole-Wheat Pizza Dough (page 229), or one 12-inch store-bought prepared pizza crust
>
> 1 cup (about 4 ounces) shredded mozzarella-style soy cheese
>
> 3 large ripe tomatoes (about $1\frac{1}{2}$ pounds), sliced $\frac{1}{4}$ inch thick
>
> 1 tablespoon olive oil
>
> $2/3$ cup grated Parmesan-style soy cheese
>
> $1/4$ cup shredded fresh basil, or 1 tablespoon dried basil

1. Heat oven to 500°F. Place oven rack in lowest position.

2. Sprinkle the bottom of a 9-inch cast-iron skillet with a little cornmeal. Spread pizza dough in the bottom of the skillet.

3. Bake until lightly browned and crisp, about 7 minutes.

4. Sprinkle half of the mozzarella over prebaked crust, leaving $\frac{1}{2}$-inch border all around. Layer tomato slices on top and drizzle with oil. Sprinkle with the remaining mozzarella and the Parmesan.

5. Return to oven and bake until topping is heated through and edge of crust is browned, 8 to 12 minutes.

6. Remove pizza from oven. Sprinkle with basil and let stand 5 minutes before cutting.

Whole-Wheat Pizza Dough

Even though this is a yeast dough, no rising is required. The secret is the initial prebaking of the crust at a high oven temperature, which causes the dough to quickly puff into a crisp crust. If you only want to make one pizza, make the whole recipe and freeze half the dough (see Make-Ahead Tip below). The whole-wheat flour contributes extra fiber and nutrients. For a lighter crust, replace 1 cup, or even just $\frac{1}{2}$ cup, of whole-wheat flour with white flour, in addition to the 1 cup of white flour that is already part of the recipe.

MAKES ENOUGH DOUGH FOR TWO 12-INCH PIZZA CRUSTS
Prep: 30 minutes / Cook: as directed in pizza recipes (page 226, 227, 228)

1 cup lukewarm water (95–105°F.)

1 envelope ($2\frac{1}{2}$ teaspoons) active dry yeast

1 teaspoon sugar

2 cups whole-wheat flour

1 cup unbleached all-purpose flour, plus extra for kneading

$\frac{1}{4}$ teaspoon salt

1 teaspoon olive oil

1. In a 1-cup glass measuring cup, stir together the water, yeast, and sugar to dissolve yeast and sugar. Let stand until foamy, 5 to 10 minutes.

2. Hand Method: In a large bowl, whisk together flours and salt. Make a well in the center. Pour yeast mixture and oil into well. Mix flour with liquid using a clean hand or a large spoon to make a soft dough. **Food Processor Method**: In a food processor, combine flours and salt with on-and-off pulses. With motor running, add yeast mixture and oil through feed tube, and continue to process just until dough comes together in a wet, sticky mass.

3. Turn dough out onto a lightly floured work surface. Knead until smooth and elastic, 5 to 10 minutes, adding flour little by little as needed to prevent sticking. Let dough rest for 10 minutes.

4. Proceed with pizza recipe.

Make-Ahead Tip: Place dough in a plastic food-storage bag, leaving a little room for expansion. Seal tightly and refrigerate for up to three days. Let return to room temperature before using. Or lightly dust dough with flour, wrap tightly in plastic wrap, and slip into freezer-proof plastic bag, and freeze for up to a month. To use, thaw in refrigerator for twelve hours or overnight. Let come to room temperature before using.

CHAPTER IX

GO-WITHS

VEGETABLES, ETC.

BROCCOLI RABE WITH GARLIC AND PARMESAN CHEESE

STIR-FRIED ORANGE BROCCOLI WITH BLACK BEAN–GARLIC SAUCE

PAN-SEARED BROCCOLI AND GARLIC

SAUTEED CABBAGE WITH RED ONION AND ORANGE

SAUTEED RED CABBAGE WITH TOMATO AND HERBS

LIMA BEANS WITH SAGE

SAUTEED LIMA BEANS AND SPINACH WITH RED BELL PEPPER

ZUCCHINI AND TOMATOES WITH SWEET POTATOES AND HERBS

STEAMED BABY CARROTS WITH FENNEL AND LEMON

STEAMED SESAME SPINACH

STEWED FENNEL WITH CARROTS AND ORANGE

ROASTED MASHED CELERY ROOT WITH MUSTARD AND GINGER

ROASTED SWEET POTATOES AND APPLES WITH CRANBERRIES

SCALLOPED CORN WITH SUN-DRIED TOMATOES

TOFU FRITTERS

GRAINS AND LEGUMES

CURRIED BROWN BASMATI RICE PILAF WITH VEGETABLES

QUINOA WITH CORN AND SCALLIONS

EDAMAME SUCCOTASH WITH SALSA

BARLEY AND EDAMAME PILAF WITH MUSHROOMS AND LEMON

JAZZED-UP CANNED BLACK BEANS

SAUCES

CHEDDAR CHEESE SAUCE

LEMON-MUSTARD SAUCE WITH HORSERADISH

FRESH TOMATO SAUCE

HOMEMADE ALL-PURPOSE TOMATO SAUCE

TOMATO-GARLIC SAUCE WITH PAPRIKA

ROASTED GARLIC SAUCE

YOGURT SCALLION SAUCE

SPICY ASIAN LIME SAUCE

CHIPOTLE MAYONNAISE

GREMOLATA

THE SIDE DISHES THAT FILL UP that little empty corner of the dinner plate are an easy way to sneak even more antioxidants and fiber into a meal, and usually with very little fat. In some cases, a vegetable side dish is easily transformed into a main dish if it's spooned over a brown-type of rice or other whole grain—a combination that improves the quality of the protein. Remember that the new dietary guidelines from the USDA recommend five to nine servings of vegetables and fruit a day, which is not as daunting as it may seem since a serving is usually about half a cup.

Produce sections in this age of super-supermarkets are practically a market in themselves, with more organic fruits and vegetables finding their way into the bins everyday. And regardless of where you live, you can usually find a seasonal farmers' market in the neighborhood.

As for frozen vegetables, the quality has improved over the last several years. If you keep the large plastic bags of frozen vegetables in your freezer, you always have them on hand for a quick side dish, soup, pasta sauce, or vegetarian main course.

The cruciferous vegetables are particularly noteworthy, given their acknowledged cancer-fighting properties. This group includes broccoli, Brussels sprouts, cauliflower, cabbage, and kale, among others. To work these into your everyday eating, there are Sauteed Cabbage with Red Onion and Orange (page 235), Pan-Seared Broccoli and Garlic (page 234), and Steamed Sesame Spinach (page 243). Many of the other vegetables in this chapter will be familiar, but they are treated in deliciously different ways: Steamed Baby Carrots with Fennel and Lemon (page 242), Lima Beans with Sage (page 238), and Stir-Fried Orange Broccoli with Black Bean–Garlic Sauce (page 233). And then there are the less familiar: Stewed Fennel with Carrots and Orange (page 244), and Roasted Mashed Celery Root with Mustard and Ginger (page 245).

For simply steamed or pan-seared vegetables, there is a selection of easy sauces for dressing them up, such as Cheddar Cheese Sauce (page 256) and Lemon-Mustard Sauce with Horseradish (page 257).

In addition to the vegetable recipes in this chapter, there is also a section devoted to side dishes made with grains and legumes, both excellent sources of protein and fiber, as well as vitamins and minerals. When it comes to grains, such as rice, bulghur, and barley, unrefined is best in order to capture the nutrients stored in the bran and germ. And as for legumes, if you have the time, cook the dried from scratch for better texture—otherwise, canned are just fine.

Broccoli Rabe with Garlic and Parmesan Cheese

Also known as broccoli rape or broccolini or rapini, this green vegetable looks as though it was on its way to becoming broccoli but didn't quite make it. But it does have all the wonderful nutritional benefits of broccoli, a cruciferous vegetable. Its pleasantly bitter taste plays well with garlic, as in this dish. If you go for the four servings, there are 5 grams of fiber and 10 grams of protein in each.

Serving Suggestions: This is perfect as a side dish with all kinds of vegetarian main courses, such as Curried Bulghur with Tomatoes and Chickpeas (page 148) or Fennel and Chickpea Stew with Apricots and Raisins (page 156). The dish also easily doubles as a pasta sauce—thin it with a little pasta cooking water and spoon it over whole-wheat spaghetti, linguine, rigatoni, or penne.

MAKES 4–6 SERVINGS
Prep: 10 minutes / Cook: 20 minutes

1 tablespoon olive oil

4 cloves garlic, thinly sliced

2 pounds broccoli rabe, tough stems removed

$\frac{1}{2}$ teaspoon salt

$\frac{1}{4}$ teaspoon crushed red pepper flakes

2 cups vegetable broth, homemade (page 101) or store-bought, or water

3 tablespoons grated Parmesan-style soy cheese

1. In a large nonstick skillet with a lid, heat oil over medium-low heat. Add garlic and cook, stirring often, until softened, 1 minute, being careful not to let garlic burn.

2. Add broccoli rabe, salt, pepper flakes, and broth. Cover the skillet tightly and simmer for 8 minutes. Uncover and continue to cook until broccoli rabe is tender and liquid has cooked off, about 7 minutes.

3. Sprinkle with Parmesan and serve at once.

Stir-Fried Orange Broccoli with Black Bean–Garlic Sauce

This takes just minutes to prepare. The bottled black bean–garlic sauce, which almost makes the broccoli seem meaty, can be found in the international or Asian food section of your supermarket. For a distinctive flavor hit in other dishes, stir a little of the black bean sauce into cooked rice or vegetables, or spoon over fish before steaming or baking.

Serving Suggestions: The broccoli makes a good companion to strongly flavored fish such as Baked Tuna with Honey Glaze and Moroccan Spices (page 190). To create a main dish, spoon the broccoli over brown basmati rice and add a carrot stick salad on the side tossed with apple juice and a little olive oil. Leftovers of this broccoli dish are even good for snacking with crackers.

MAKES 4 SERVINGS
Prep: 10 minutes / Cook: 6 minutes

2 tablespoons light olive oil
1 medium-size head broccoli, top separated into small florets, and stems peeled and cut into thin coins
$\frac{1}{2}$ cup orange juice
1 tablespoon grated orange zest
2 teaspoons bottled black bean–garlic sauce

1. In a large nonstick skillet with a lid, heat oil over medium-high heat. Add broccoli and stir-fry for 3 minutes. Add $\frac{1}{4}$ cup of the orange juice, cover, and simmer until crisp-tender, about 2 minutes.

2. Add the remaining $\frac{1}{4}$ cup orange juice, zest, and black bean sauce and stir-fry until broccoli is well coated and most liquid has been absorbed, about 30 seconds. Serve immediately.

Make-Ahead Tip: Cooked broccoli can be refrigerated for up to a day. Gently reheat in a skillet or microwave.

Pan-Seared Broccoli and Garlic

This flavorful way to cook broccoli also works well for cauliflower, asparagus, carrots, and green beans. A large, well-seasoned cast-iron skillet works best, but any heavy-duty skillet will be okay. Cooking times will vary according to the quantity of the vegetable and the vegetable itself: asparagus cooks faster than broccoli, and carrots take a little longer than broccoli. Also, keep the pieces small and equal in size so they cook uniformly. Experiment with different liquids for the cooking, for a variety of tastes.

Serving Suggestions: Just before removing the cooked broccoli from the skillet, sprinkle it with Parmesan-style soy cheese. Add leftover broccoli to salads, or munch as is for a healthy, flavorful snack.

MAKES 4 SERVINGS
Prep: 10 minutes / Cook: about 15 minutes

- 1 tablespoon olive oil
- 4 cloves garlic, thinly sliced
- 1 head broccoli, top separated into small florets, and stems trimmed, peeled, and cut into thin coins
- $\frac{1}{4}$ cup vegetable broth, homemade (page 101) or store-bought, or orange juice, or apple juice

1. In a large cast-iron skillet with a lid, heat oil over medium heat. Add garlic and cook, stirring frequently, for 1 minute, being careful not to let garlic burn.
2. Add broccoli and cook, turning pieces over frequently, for 2 minutes.
3. Add broth, cover the skillet, and cook until crisp-tender, 8 to 10 minutes.

Make-Ahead Tip: Broccoli can be refrigerated for up to a day. Reheat it in a skillet or microwave.

Sauteed Cabbage with Red Onion and Orange

This is an easy dish to toss together, and it tastes good seasoned either with cumin or caraway, depending on your own likes. Of course, cabbage, a cruciferous vegetable, provides a variety of phytochemicals that may help to protect against cancer.

Serving Suggestions: To use the cabbage mixture in a sandwich melt, spread Dijon mustard on slices of toasted whole-grain bread, pile on the cabbage mixture, top with slices of Monterey Jack–style or cheddar-style soy cheese, and heat in a microwave or run under a broiler to melt the cheese. To stuff a whole bread loaf using the cabbage mixture as the stuffing, see page 86. On its own, serve the cabbage with Broiled Tuna with Horseradish and Apple (page 204) or other strong-flavored fish, or with Nutty Lentil Loaf with Veggies and Mozzarella Cheese (page 158). The cabbage mixture also makes a crunchy salad if served at room temperature or chilled.

MAKES 6 SERVINGS
Prep: 10 minutes / Cook: 10 minutes

2 tablespoons olive oil

1 small red onion, halved and cut crosswise into thin half moons

3 cloves garlic, finely chopped

1 small head green cabbage (about 2 pounds), halved, cored, and thinly shredded

1 tablespoon ground cumin or caraway seeds, crushed

$\frac{1}{2}$ teaspoon salt

$\frac{1}{4}$ teaspoon black pepper

$\frac{1}{2}$ cup orange juice

1 tablespoon grated orange zest

1. In a large nonstick skillet, heat oil over medium heat. Add onion and cook, stirring occasionally, until softened, about 4 minutes. Add garlic and cook for 1 minute.

2. Add cabbage, cumin or caraway, salt, pepper, and orange juice and cook, stirring frequently, until cabbage is crisp-tender, 5 to 8 minutes. Stir in zest, and serve.

Make-Ahead Tip: Cabbage mixture can be refrigerated for up to two days. Gently reheat it or serve it chilled or at room temperature.

Sauteed Red Cabbage with Tomato and Herbs

This recipe was taught to me by a very good friend, Stephen Frankel, who based it on a Jewish-Romanian dish his mother made frequently while he was growing up. Stephen prepares it by taste and watching it as it cooks, with no written recipe to follow. For me to duplicate it, he had to cook me the dish while I watched and frantically took notes.

The trick is to very thinly slice the cabbage and to cook the cabbage mixture slowly so the final dish is thick, with just the slightest hint of crunch. This dish seems to have a better flavor if not cooked in a nonstick pot. Although the lengthy stove-top cooking requires your attention, the payoff is a deliciously textured dish that keeps well in the refrigerator for a few days so you can have it on hand.

In addition to the beneficial phytochemicals with known disease-fighting capabilities common to all cabbages, red cabbage also contains anthocyanins that fight inflammation and protect blood vessels. The tomato is a good source of lycopene and cooking it with olive oil makes it more bioavailable.

Serving Suggestions: Spoon the cabbage over mashed potatoes or Roasted Mashed Celery Root with Mustard and Ginger (page 245) for a vegetarian main dish, and accompany with a shredded carrot salad. The cabbage also pairs well with fish, such as Yogurt-Mustard Cod Fillets with Dill (page 206). And, you can serve it at room temperature as a salad with a sandwich such as Sweet Potato Burger with Kale and Black-Eyed Peas (page 89).

MAKES 6 SERVINGS
Prep: 15 minutes / Cook: 35 minutes

> 3 tablespoons olive oil
>
> 1 small yellow onion, cut into small dice (about 2 cups)
>
> 1 small red cabbage (about $1\frac{1}{2}$ pounds), cored and very thinly shredded (about 8 cups)
>
> 2 to 3 teaspoon herbes de Provence (see Note below)
>
> 2 teaspoons sugar
>
> 1 tablespoon tomato paste
>
> 1 can (8 ounces) tomato sauce
>
> $\frac{1}{2}$ teaspoon salt
>
> $\frac{1}{4}$ teaspoon black pepper

1. In a large saucepan or pot, heat 2 tablespoons of the oil over medium heat. Add onion and reduce heat to low. Partially cover pan and cook, stirring occasionally, until onion is softened and very lightly colored, about 8 minutes. Remove the pan from heat and let stand for 5 minutes. Transfer onion to small bowl.

2. Add remaining tablespoon of oil to pan and heat. Add cabbage and stir to coat with oil. Partially cover pan and cook, stirring occasionally, until cabbage begins to wilt but is still slightly crunchy, 5 to 8 minutes. Stir in 1 teaspoon of the herbs, the sugar, and a tablespoon or two of water if cabbage is sticking to the pan. Partially cover the pan and cook, stirring occasionally, until cabbage is very tender, 10 to 12 minutes.

3. Stir onion into cabbage and cook, covered, for 1 minute. Stir in tomato paste, tomato sauce, remaining herbs, salt, and pepper. Cook, covered, over low heat to blend flavors and heat through, stirring frequently, about 5 minutes.

Make-Ahead: Cabbage mixture can be refrigerated for up to three days.

Note: Herbes de Provence is an herb blend that can be found in the spice section of better supermarkets. Or make your own: Use a mortar and pestle or the back of a spoon in a metal bowl to grind together 1 tablespoon dried thyme, 1 teaspoon dried basil, 1 teaspoon dried rosemary, and $\frac{1}{4}$ teaspoon fennel seeds. Store in an airtight container in a cool, dark place for up to six months.

Lima Beans with Sage

You need four ingredients for this easy side dish—that's it! Limas are a good source of antioxidants and supply about 6 grams of protein per $\frac{1}{2}$-cup serving, with no fat. You can substitute frozen peas for the limas.

Serving Suggestions: Serve with grain dishes such as Barley Risotto with Asparagus and Mushrooms (page 145) or Smoky Cheese Enchiladas (page 171), or a simple fish dish such as Scrod with Corn and Tomato (page 202). To quickly transform leftover limas into a simple protein-rich side salad, sprinkle with a little balsamic vinegar and finely chopped scallions.

MAKES 4 SERVINGS
Prep: 5 minutes / Cook: 15 minutes

> 2 cups frozen lima beans, or frozen peas
> 1 tablespoon olive oil
> 2 teaspoons dried sage
> $\frac{1}{8}$ teaspoon salt

1. In a small saucepan, cook lima beans according to package directions. Drain and return to the saucepan.

2. Stir in oil to coat limas. Stir in sage and salt and serve.

Sauteed Lima Beans and Spinach with Red Bell Pepper

Lima beans are meaty tasting and, perhaps more important, a nutritional powerhouse, providing protein and fiber as well as iron and potassium. In this recipe, the protein registers at 7 grams per serving, and the fiber is an amazing 9 grams. Antioxidants show up in the red bell pepper and spinach. And the combination of fennel and sage strikes a bass note on the palate.

Serving Suggestions: The lima bean combination is a tasty complement to Spinach-Corn Couscous with Baked Tofu (page 152). It's also easily transformed into a pasta dish (page 218). Toss the mixture with a little extra-virgin olive oil and balsamic vinegar and serve it at room temperature as a salad.

MAKES 4 SERVINGS
Prep: 5 minutes / Cook: 7 minutes

2 tablespoons olive oil

2 cloves garlic, finely chopped

1 red bell pepper, cored, seeded, and chopped

$\frac{3}{4}$ teaspoon ground fennel

$\frac{1}{2}$ teaspoon dried sage

$\frac{1}{4}$ teaspoon salt

1 box (10 ounces) frozen lima beans, thawed (about 2 cups)

1 bag (about 9 ounces) fresh baby spinach

1. In a large nonstick pot or skillet, heat oil over medium heat. Add garlic and bell pepper and cook, stirring, occasionally, until softened, about 3 minutes. Stir in fennel, sage, salt, and lima beans and cook, stirring, for 2 minutes.

2. Add spinach and cook, stirring, until wilted and lima beans are heated through, about 2 minutes. Serve immediately.

Make-Ahead Tip: Lima bean mixture can be refrigerated for up to two days. Gently reheat it in a skillet or serve it at room temperature.

Zucchini and Tomatoes with Sweet Potatoes and Herbs

Based on the Mediterranean dish ratatouille, my take on this combination of vegetables also includes the antioxidant-rich sweet potato, which I've substituted for the usual eggplant. The recipe makes a large quantity so there are lots of leftovers for all the serving suggestions that follow, or you can store some in the freezer.

Serving Suggestions: Serve bowls of this with Broiled Salmon with Cumin and Lemon (page 192) or Jimmy's Baltimore Salmon Cakes (page 194), or with grain dishes such as Curried Bulghur with Tomatoes and Chickpeas (page 148) or Barley with Black Beans and Roasted Peppers (page 146). For a quick salad, you can serve the zucchini mixture at room temperature. For a pasta salad, stir in cooled, cooked whole-grain rigatoni or penne.

MAKES 12 SERVINGS
Prep: 15 minutes / Cook: 50 minutes

> 3 tablespoons olive oil
>
> 2 sweet onions such as Vidalia, chopped
>
> 2 cloves garlic, finely chopped
>
> 3 green bell peppers, or a combination of different colored peppers, cored, seeded, and cut into small dice
>
> 4 medium-size zucchini, trimmed and thinly sliced
>
> 2 medium-size sweet potatoes (about 1 pound), peeled and cut into $\frac{1}{2}$-inch cubes
>
> 1 can (32 ounces) whole tomatoes, chopped
>
> 1 teaspoon dried basil
>
> 1 teaspoon dried oregano
>
> $\frac{1}{2}$ teaspoon salt
>
> $\frac{1}{4}$ teaspoon black pepper
>
> 2 tablespoons balsamic or red-wine vinegar (optional)
>
> $\frac{1}{4}$ cup chopped fresh parsley

1. In a large nonstick pot, heat oil over medium heat. Add onions and cook, stirring occasionally, until slightly softened, about 5 minutes. Stir in garlic and cook for 1 minute.
2. Add bell peppers and cook, stirring occasionally, until slightly softened, about 4 minutes. Add zucchini and cook for 4 minutes. Add sweet potatoes and cook for 4 more minutes.
3. Stir in tomatoes with their liquid, basil, oregano, salt, pepper, and vinegar if using, and bring to a boil. Lower heat and simmer, covered, until sweet potatoes are firm-tender,

about 30 minutes. Uncover and check the consistency—mixture should be thick. If it's too liquidy, gently boil until some of the liquid cooks off.

4. Stir in parsley just before serving.

Make-Ahead Tip: The mixture, without the parsley, can be refrigerated for up to three days, or frozen for up to a month. Stir in parsley just before serving.

Steamed Baby Carrots with Fennel and Lemon

Beta-carotene is the star antioxidant in carrots. For this dish, which is very quick to make, you can substitute other dried herbs for the fennel—basil, tarragon, marjoram, thyme, or rosemary—and orange for the lemon.

Serving Suggestions: This dish works well anywhere you would usually serve carrots. And, like many side dishes in this chapter, it makes a crunchy vegetable side salad if served chilled or at room temperature.

MAKES 6 SERVINGS
Prep: 5 minutes / Cook: 8 minutes

> 2 bags (12 ounces each) baby carrots
>
> 2 tablespoons olive oil
>
> $\frac{1}{2}$ teaspoon grated lemon zest, or orange zest
>
> 2 teaspoons freshly squeezed lemon juice, or more to taste, or orange juice
>
> 1 tablespoon fennel seeds, lightly crushed
>
> $\frac{1}{4}$ teaspoon salt
>
> $\frac{1}{8}$ teaspoon black pepper

1. In a steamer or medium-size saucepan fitted with a steamer basket over simmering water, steam carrots, covered, until tender, about 8 minutes.

2. Transfer carrots to a bowl. Add oil, lemon zest and juice, fennel, salt, and pepper, and toss to coat carrots well. Serve.

Make-Ahead Tip: Carrots can be refrigerated for up to three days and reheated in a skillet, or served chilled or at room temperature as a salad.

Steamed Sesame Spinach

Fresh organic spinach from a farmers' market is the best bet for this dish, but for convenience, you can purchase packaged, prewashed organic spinach from the supermarket. Spinach is considered a superfood by some since it contains a wealth of phytonutrients, antioxidants, minerals, and even plant-derived omega-3 fatty acids. Adding star anise (see Note below) or whole cloves to the steaming water imparts a subtle flavor to the dish.

Serving Suggestions: Cooked in 5 minutes, the spinach makes an easily prepared accent to Baked Sea Bass with Tomato and Black Olives (page 191) or Soy-Glazed Halibut with Shiitake Mushrooms (page 207).

MAKES 4 SERVINGS
Prep: 10 minutes / Cook: 5 minutes

> 2 star anise (see Note below), or 2 whole cloves
>
> 1 pound fresh spinach, cleaned and tough stems removed
>
> $\frac{1}{8}$ teaspoon crushed red pepper flakes
>
> $\frac{1}{2}$ teaspoon dark sesame oil
>
> 1 teaspoon salt
>
> 1 teaspoon freshly squeezed lemon juice
>
> 1 tablespoon sesame seeds, toasted (see Note below)

1. Fill a steamer or saucepan fitted with a steamer basket, with about 1 inch of water, add star anise or whole cloves, cover, and bring to a boil. Carefully add spinach and pepper flakes to the steamer basket. Cover the pot and steam until spinach is tender but not overly wilted, 2 to 3 minutes. Transfer to a serving bowl.

2. Add sesame oil, salt, and lemon juice and toss to mix. Sprinkle with sesame seeds and serve immediately.

Note: In a small, dry skillet, toast sesame seeds over medium heat until lightly colored, 2 to 3 minutes. Watch carefully—they burn quickly.

Star anise is a small, six- to eight-pointed starlike pod that comes from a tree belonging to the magnolia family and is grown in northern Vietnam and southern China. This spice is often used to infuse cooking broths or steaming liquids with its distinctive licorice flavor, which also has cinnamon and clove overtones. If using the pods in a stew, be sure to remove them before serving as you would bay leaves or whole cloves.

Stewed Fennel with Carrots and Orange

The carrots and the orange contribute lots of antioxidants. This vegetable dish has a bright, sunny flavor, with hints of licorice or anise from the fresh fennel. Fennel, which is crunchy like celery, is usually available year round in the supermarket. You can thinly slice the stalks and toss them into salad.

Serving Suggestions: Serve with a mild-tasting fish such as cod, haddock, or halibut. For a main dish, spoon over brown basmati rice or other brown rice, or whole-wheat noodles. This dish is even tasty at room temperature or slightly chilled as a salad.

MAKES 4 SERVINGS

Prep: 15 minutes / Cook: about 30 minutes

2 teaspoons olive oil

1 sweet onion such as Vidalia, finely chopped

2 cloves garlic, finely chopped

1 teaspoon dried rosemary, crumbled

1 strip orange zest

$\frac{1}{2}$ teaspoon salt

1 bulb fresh fennel with stalks

$\frac{1}{2}$ pound carrots, trimmed, peeled, and cut into $\frac{1}{4}$-inch-thick slices

$\frac{1}{4}$ cup orange juice

1. In a large nonstick skillet, heat oil over medium heat. Add onion, garlic, rosemary, orange zest, and salt, and cook, stirring frequently, until onion is lightly browned and very soft, about 8 minutes.

2. Meanwhile, remove feathery fronds from fennel and save for soup or seasoning other dishes. Cut stalks from bulb and thinly slice stalks. Cut bulb in half and remove core. Cut bulb into $\frac{1}{2}$-inch-thick wedges.

3. Add fennel, carrots, and orange juice to skillet, stirring to combine. Bring to a boil. Reduce heat, cover skillet tightly, and simmer until carrots and fennel are tender, 15 to 20 minutes.

Make-Ahead Tip: Stewed fennel can be prepared up to two days ahead and refrigerated. Rewarm it in a skillet or microwave.

Roasted Mashed Celery Root with Mustard and Ginger

Celery root, with a subtle celery flavor, is an unattractive but delicious root vegetable that's in the markets from fall through winter. When roasted and mashed, it makes an intriguing alternative to the usual mashed white potatoes and boosts the fiber—there are 5 grams per serving in this dish. The tamari and fresh ginger give this dish an Asian flavor. Notice that the prep time is short while the cooking time is long—that's unattended roasting time, so you're not chained to the stove. Plus, the puree can be made a day ahead.

Serving Suggestions: This would be an unusual but tasty counterpoint to broiled bluefish, salmon, or haddock, or as a side with a saucy vegetarian main dish, such as Chickpeas with Squash and Tomatoes (page 166) or Red Lentil and Sweet Potato Stew with Indian Spices (page 168), or with another saucy side dish, such as Zucchini and Tomatoes with Sweet Potatoes and Herbs (page 240) or Sauteed Lima Beans and Spinach with Red Bell Pepper (page 239). Leftover mashed celery root can be shaped into patties, coated in rice flour or whole-wheat flour, and then pan-fried in a nonstick skillet coated with nonstick olive oil cooking spray.

MAKES 4 SERVINGS
Prep: 10 minutes / Cook: $1\frac{1}{2}$ hours.

> 2 medium-size celery roots ($1\frac{1}{4}$–$1\frac{1}{2}$ pounds each), scrubbed and with skin left on
> Light olive oil
> 1–2 tablespoons Dijon mustard
> 1–2 tablespoons tamari or soy sauce
> 1 tablespoon peeled, finely chopped fresh ginger
> $\frac{1}{4}$ teaspoon black pepper
> $\frac{1}{4}$ cup vegetable broth, homemade (page 101) or store-bought, heated

1. Heat oven to 350°F. Generously rub celery root with oil. Place on a baking pan.

2. Bake until very tender, about $1\frac{1}{2}$ hours.

3. While celery root is hot, peel off rough skin with a knife. Cut root into small pieces. Place in a food processor. Add mustard, tamari, ginger, and pepper. Process until mashed, adding broth as needed to adjust consistency. Serve hot.

Make-Ahead Tip: Mashed celery root can be refrigerated for up to two days. Gently reheat in a saucepan, stirring. Add more broth or a little unsweetened soy milk for a fluffier mixture.

Roasted Sweet Potatoes and Apples with Cranberries

There are so many antioxidants in this dish. It's worth freezing bags of cranberries when they're abundantly available in the fall, since this is actually very good as a cold salad in the summer. But if you can't get your hands on cranberries in the summer, you can substitute about $\frac{1}{2}$ cup chopped dried apricots or raisins or dried cranberries.

Serving Suggestions: This would be yummy with Chickpea and Spinach Loaf with Mustard-Ketchup Topping (page 160), or as a cold salad, almost like potato salad, with sandwiches for lunch, or with Pumpkin Pancakes (page 275) for breakfast.

MAKES 8 SERVINGS
Prep: 10 minutes / Cook: 30 minutes

> Nonstick olive oil cooking spray
> 3 medium-size sweet potatoes (about 1 pound), peeled, halved lengthwise, and cut crosswise into $\frac{1}{4}$-inch-thick slices
> 1 tablespoon light olive oil
> 4 Granny Smith or other crisp apples, peeled, halved, cored, and each half cut into 4 wedges
> $\frac{1}{3}$ cup maple syrup
> $\frac{3}{4}$ teaspoon ground cinnamon
> $\frac{1}{4}$ teaspoon ground cloves
> $\frac{1}{8}$ teaspoon ground nutmeg
> $\frac{1}{4}$ teaspoon salt
> $1\frac{1}{2}$ cups cranberries

1. Heat oven to 425°F. Lightly coat a roasting pan, large broiler pan bottom, or large baking pan with cooking spray. The pan needs to be large enough to hold sweet potato pieces in a single layer.

2. In a large bowl, toss together sweet potatoes and oil to coat potatoes. Spread in a single layer in the prepared pan.

3. Roast for 15 minutes, carefully stirring halfway through.

4. Remove the pan from the oven. Add apples to potatoes. Drizzle with syrup, and sprinkle with cinnamon, cloves, nutmeg, and salt. Carefully stir to evenly coat, without breaking apple or potato pieces.

5. Return the pan to the oven and roast until potatoes are crisp-tender, about 10 minutes, stirring halfway through.

6. Remove the pan from the oven. Add cranberries and gently stir to mix.

7. Return to the oven until cranberries are softened and all other ingredients are tender, about 5 minutes. Let stand 5 minutes before serving.

Make-Ahead Tip: Sweet potato mixture can be refrigerated for up to three days and reheated in a 350°F oven or in a large nonstick skillet. Or serve chilled or at room temperature as a salad.

Scalloped Corn with Sun-Dried Tomatoes

An old-fashioned favorite redone. Using soy milk eliminates the cholesterol usually found in this dish and reduces the fat, and the sun-dried tomatoes add a sweet-tart flavor as well as lycopene.

Serving Suggestions: For an easy casserole dinner, serve as a side dish with any of the casseroles in the Vegetarian Main Dishes chapter (page 142), or with Jimmy's Baltimore Salmon Cakes (page 194), or with Cod in Tomato-Ginger Sauce (page 198). Or you could create a buffet with other side dishes such as Zucchini and Tomatoes with Sweet Potatoes and Herbs (page 240) or Barley and Edamame Pilaf with Mushrooms and Lemon (page 254).

MAKES 6 SERVINGS

Prep: 10 minutes / Cook: about 40 minutes

   2 tablespoons olive oil

   1 cup chopped scallions (about 1 bunch)

   $\frac{1}{2}$ cup oil-packed sun-dried tomatoes, drained on paper towels and chopped

   2 tablespoons unbleached white flour or brown rice flour

   1 tablespoon Dijon mustard

   $1\frac{1}{2}$ cups unsweetened soy milk

   3 cups frozen corn kernels, thawed

   $\frac{1}{2}$ teaspoon dried thyme

   $\frac{1}{2}$ teaspoon salt

   $\frac{1}{4}$ teaspoon black pepper

   1 cup whole-grain bread crumbs (from about 1 slice)

1. Heat oven to 350°F.

2. In a large nonstick skillet, heat $1\frac{1}{2}$ tablespoons of the oil over medium heat. Add scallions and cook, stirring occasionally, until softened and lightly colored, 3 to 5 minutes. Add sun-dried tomatoes and cook, stirring occasionally, for 1 minute.

3. Sprinkle flour over scallion mixture and cook, stirring, for 1 minute. Stir in mustard until thoroughly combined. Gradually stir in soy milk until well blended. Add corn and thyme. Cook, stirring, until thickened, about 1 to 2 minutes. Stir in salt and pepper. Scrape into a 13 x 9 x 2-inch glass baking dish.

4. In a small bowl, stir together bread crumbs and the remaining $\frac{1}{2}$ tablespoon oil. Scatter evenly over top of casserole.

5. Bake until topping is browned and crisped and filling is bubbly, about 30 minutes. Let stand for 10 minutes.

Make-Ahead Tip: Unbaked casserole without bread topping can be made a day ahead and refrigerated. Let come to room temperature, sprinkle with bread crumbs, and bake as directed above. Leftovers can be reheated in a microwave or 350°F oven.

Tofu Fritters

Grated carrots add an extra boost of antioxidants to this fun fritter, and the white rice creates a soft texture, although brown basmati can be substituted. You can use regular flour to coat the outside of the fritters or, for a slightly crisper coating, try brown rice flour.

Serving Suggestions: These are delicious on their own as a snack, as a party nibble, or as part of a brunch buffet. As a side dish they can be served plain or with Homemade All-Purpose Tomato Sauce (page 259), then paired with Red Lentil and Sweet Potato Stew with Indian Spices (page 168), Curried Vegetable Stew with Coconut (page 184), or Curried Bulghur with Tomatoes and Chickpeas (page 148).

MAKES 8 FRITTERS

Prep: 15 minutes / Cook: about 6 minutes per batch.

> 1 box (12.3 ounces) silken firm tofu
> 1 cup cooked white or brown basmati rice
> 2 scallions, trimmed and finely chopped
> 1 medium-size carrot, trimmed, peeled, and finely grated
> 1 tablespoon sesame seeds
> 1 tablespoon regular or reduced-sodium soy sauce
> 1 tablespoon all-purpose flour, or whole-wheat flour
> $\frac{1}{2}$ teaspoon salt
> $\frac{1}{8}$ teaspoon black pepper
> All-purpose flour or brown rice flour, for coating
> 2 tablespoons light olive oil

1. In a medium-size bowl, mash tofu. Stir in cooked rice, scallions, carrot, sesame seeds, soy sauce, 1 tablespoon flour, salt, and pepper.

2. Shape mixture into 8 equal-size balls and flatten to form patties. Coat patties with flour.

3. In a large nonstick skillet, heat oil over medium heat. Add 2 or 3 patties to the pan and cook until lightly browned, about 3 minutes. Turn over and brown other side, about 3 minutes. Remove to a plate and cover to keep warm. Repeat with remaining patties. Serve hot.

Curried Brown Basmati Rice Pilaf with Vegetables

Instead of plain white rice, this recipe calls for the more nutrient- and fiber-rich brown basmati rice. Some of the individual spices that make up curry powder may contain prostate cancer-fighting properties. Brazil nuts are a good source of selenium.

Serving Suggestions: The spicy pilaf goes well with Halibut with Orange-Ginger Sauce (page 199) or with a piece of plain broiled fish. To easily convert the pilaf into a main course, add Greek-Style Marinated Tofu (page 66). To create a salad, stir a little mango chutney into the pilaf and serve it chilled or at room temperature.

MAKES 8 SERVINGS

Prep: 10 minutes / Cook: 55 minutes

- 2 tablespoons light olive oil
- 1 large onion, thinly sliced
- 2 teaspoons curry powder
- 1½ cups brown basmati rice
- ¼ cup golden raisins
- 1 cinnamon stick
- 3 cups vegetable broth, homemade (page 101) or store-bought
- 1 red bell pepper, cored, seeded, and thinly sliced
- 1 carrot, trimmed, peeled, and shredded
- ½ cup frozen peas, or frozen corn kernels
- ¼ cup Brazil nuts, coarsely chopped

1. In a large skillet, heat oil over medium heat. Add onion and cook, stirring occasionally, until lightly golden, about 6 minutes. Stir in curry powder and rice. Stir in raisins, cinnamon stick, and broth. Bring to a boil. Lower heat, cover, and simmer for 40 minutes.

2. Stir in bell pepper and carrot. Cover and simmer for 5 minutes. Stir in peas. Remove the skillet from heat and let stand, covered, for 10 minutes.

3. Meanwhile, in a medium-size dry skillet, toast nuts over medium heat until lightly browned, about 2 minutes. Remove from heat.

4. To serve, remove cinnamon stick from rice, and sprinkle nuts over top.

Make-Ahead Tip: Rice can be prepared up to two days ahead and refrigerated, and then reheated in a saucepan or microwave, adding broth or water as needed.

Quinoa with Corn and Scallions

Quinoa (*keen*-wah) was one of the main sources of protein for the ancient Incas of the Andes. Even though it looks and tastes like one, it is not really a grain, but rather the fruit of an herb. Quinoa is more protein-rich than any grain, and it is a complete protein—it contains all eight essential amino acids. And it doesn't stop there. Quinoa is higher in unsaturated fats than any grain. It is important to rinse quinoa very well, for at least a minute or two, to remove the natural coating, saponin, which has a slightly bitter, soapy taste. Toasting it in a dry skillet over medium heat for a minute or two adds a nutty, sweet flavor. Quinoa is delicious on its own, prepared by following the package directions. This recipe shows you how to jazz it up.

Serving Suggestions: Serve with vegetarian main dishes such as Fennel and Chickpea Stew with Apricots and Raisins (page 156) or Chickpeas with Squash and Tomatoes (page 166), or with another vegetable side dish such as Lima Beans with Sage (page 238), or even with fish such as Haddock Fillets with Blood Oranges and Mustard (page 205). Chilled quinoa leftovers, tossed with a mild-tasting rice vinegar, spooned over a bed of spinach or other dark leafy greens, and accompanied with a whole-grain bread, makes an easy lunch.

MAKES 6 SERVINGS

Prep: 10 minutes / Cook: about 15 minutes

> 1 cup quinoa, very well rinsed and drained
>
> 2 cups vegetable broth, homemade (page 101) or store-bought, or water
>
> $\frac{1}{2}$ teaspoon salt
>
> 2 cups frozen corn kernels
>
> 5 scallions, trimmed and finely chopped
>
> $\frac{1}{4}$ cup chopped fresh flat-leaf parsley, or fresh basil

1. Blot quinoa dry with paper towels. Heat a large, dry nonstick skillet over medium heat. Add quinoa and toast, stirring frequently, until grains are dry and some begin to pop, 3 to 4 minutes.

2. In a medium-size saucepan, bring broth and salt to a boil. Add quinoa and stir. Cover pan, reduce heat, and simmer for 12 minutes. Stir in corn and scallions. Simmer, covered, until quinoa is firm but tender, another 3 to 4 minutes. All the liquid should be absorbed and "grains" should have opened up into tiny star shapes. Remove from heat and let stand, covered, 5 minutes.

3. Fluff with fork, stirring in parsley, and serve.

Make-Ahead Tip: Quinoa can be made a day ahead, without parsley, and refrigerated. Reheat by steaming or microwaving, adding a little vegetable broth or water if mixture appears too dry, and then stir in parsley.

Edamame Succotash with Salsa

Even though this is a side dish, since the edamame pack a protein wallop (8 grams per serving, along with 5 grams of fiber), the addition of a little cooked brown rice would easily convert this go-with to a main dish. The salsa adds a shot of lycopene.

Serving Suggestions: The succotash would deliciously complement Broiled Cod with Sun-Dried Tomato Sauce (page 200). And if you serve the succotash at room temperature or chilled, it becomes a vegetable salad that makes a tasty accompaniment to sandwiches.

MAKES 4 SERVINGS
Prep: 5 minutes / Cook: 5 minutes

$1\frac{1}{2}$ cups frozen shelled and blanched edamame

1 can (15 ounces) whole-kernel corn, drained and rinsed, or 2 cups frozen corn kernels

$\frac{1}{4}$ cup vegetable broth, homemade (page 101) or store-bought

$\frac{1}{4}$ cup bottled medium-hot salsa

$\frac{3}{4}$ teaspoon dried oregano

$\frac{1}{4}$ teaspoon salt

$\frac{1}{8}$ teaspoon black pepper

In a medium-size nonstick saucepan, stir together edamame, corn, vegetable broth, salsa, oregano, salt, and pepper. Simmer over medium-high heat until heated through, about 5 minutes.

Make-Ahead Tip: Succotash can be refrigerated for up to three days. Gently rewarm in a saucepan.

Barley and Edamame Pilaf with Mushrooms and Lemon

Here's another way to introduce edamame, with its high-quality protein, into your diet. The edamame combines with the barley and mushrooms for a very satisfying taste. A flavor trick is to first toast the barley.

Serving Suggestions: Use as an accompaniment for one of the burgers in the sandwich chapter or with Broiled Salmon with Cumin and Lemon (page 192) or other simple fish dishes. To create a salad from the leftovers, sprinkle it with a little balsamic vinegar and top with crumbled feta-style soy cheese.

MAKES 6 SERVINGS

Prep: 15 minutes / Cook: about 40 minutes

$\frac{3}{4}$ cup pearl barley

1 tablespoon light olive oil

1 large onion, chopped

2 cups vegetable broth, homemade (page 101) or store-bought

1 cup coarsely chopped baby bella mushrooms, or white button mushrooms

$\frac{3}{4}$ teaspoon dried thyme

1 cup frozen shelled and blanched edamame

1 small red bell pepper, cored, seeded, and chopped

1 teaspoon grated lemon zest

$\frac{1}{2}$ teaspoon salt

$\frac{1}{4}$ teaspoon black pepper

1. In a medium-size dry nonstick saucepan, cook barley over medium heat, stirring frequently, until fragrant and golden, stirring constantly toward end of cooking, 4 to 5 minutes. Scrape barley into small bowl and set aside.

2. In the same saucepan, heat oil over medium heat. Add onion and cook, stirring occasionally, until softened, about 6 minutes. Stir in broth, mushrooms, thyme, and reserved barley. Bring to a simmer. Reduce heat to low and cook, covered, until barley is almost tender, about 25 minutes.

3. Stir in edamame, bell pepper, lemon zest, salt, and pepper. Cook, covered, until barley and vegetables are tender, about 6 minutes. Serve hot.

Make-Ahead Tip: Pilaf can be made a day ahead and refrigerated. Gently reheat it in a saucepan or in the microwave, adding broth or water as needed if it appears too dry.

Jazzed-Up Canned Black Beans

Here's an easy way to add a little extra zip to canned black beans. And remember, black beans kick in fiber and protein—6 grams fiber and 5 grams protein per serving for this dish.

Serving Suggestions: Spoon the beans over brown rice or whole-wheat couscous, top with shredded jalapeño Jack–style soy cheese or cheddar-style soy cheese, and you have a main course. Or couple as a side dish with a grain main dish such as Baked Rice and Jack Cheese Casserole with Chiles and Corn (page 144). These beans are good even on their own with homemade (page 55) or store-bought baked tortilla chips. Pair with a salad, and you have lunch or a light supper.

MAKES 6 SERVINGS
Prep: 10 minutes / Cook: about 25 minutes

> 1 tablespoon olive oil
> 1 small sweet onion such as Vidalia, chopped
> 2 cloves garlic, finely chopped
> $\frac{1}{2}$ of red bell pepper, cored, seeded, and chopped
> 2 cans (15 ounces each) black beans, drained and rinsed
> 1 teaspoon ground cumin
> $\frac{1}{4}$ teaspoon salt
> $\frac{1}{4}$ teaspoon black pepper
> $\frac{1}{2}$ cup vegetable broth, homemade (page 101) or store-bought
> 1 tablespoon freshly squeezed lime or lemon juice

1. In a large nonstick saucepan, heat oil over medium heat. Add onion and cook, stirring occasionally, until softened, about 5 minutes. Stir in garlic and bell pepper, and cook, stirring occasionally, until pepper is softened, about 5 minutes.

2. Stir in beans, cumin, salt, pepper, and broth. With a potato masher or the back of a spoon, mash about one-quarter of the beans. Bring to a simmer and cook for 15 minutes.

3. Stir in lime juice just before serving.

Make-Ahead Tip: Leftovers can be refrigerated for up to three days, or frozen for up to a month. If you're making the whole batch ahead of time, omit lime juice and stir it in just before serving.

Cheddar Cheese Sauce

Accented with Dijon mustard, this rich sauce derives its creaminess from silken tofu.

Serving Suggestions: Spoon over steamed broccoli, or asparagus, or other cooked vegetables, or over mashed Yukon gold potatoes.

MAKES ABOUT $2\frac{1}{4}$ CUPS
Prep: 5 minutes / Cook: 2 minutes

1 box (12.3 ounces) silken soft tofu
$\frac{1}{2}$ cup unsweetened soy milk
1 package (7 ounces) shredded cheddar-style soy cheese (about $1\frac{3}{4}$ cups)
2 teaspoons Dijon mustard
$\frac{1}{2}$ teaspoon dried tarragon

1. In a blender or small food processor, puree together tofu and soy milk until smooth. Pour into saucepan.

2. Stir in cheese and mustard and gently heat over medium-low heat, stirring, until cheese melts and sauce is smooth, about 2 minutes. Stir in tarragon.

Make-Ahead Tip: Sauce can be refrigerated for up to three days. Gently reheat in a saucepan.

Lemon-Mustard Sauce with Horseradish

The flavors of the lemon, mustard, and horseradish play off of each other very well. This recipe is enough for four servings of vegetable—it coats the vegetables rather than saucing them.

Serving Suggestions: Toss with broccoli, cauliflower, Brussels sprouts, peas, green beans, or carrots, or spoon over cod, haddock, or halibut.

MAKES $\frac{1}{4}$ CUP
Prep: 5 minutes / Cook: 2 minutes

   2 tablespoons Dijon mustard

   2 teaspoons olive oil

   2 teaspoons grated lemon zest

   1 teaspoon freshly squeezed lemon juice

   1 teaspoon bottled horseradish, drained

1. In a small nonstick saucepan, stir together all the ingredients.

2. Place over low heat and gently heat through, stirring occasionally, without boiling.

Make-Ahead Tip: Sauce can be refrigerated for up to a day. Gently reheat, without boiling.

Fresh Tomato Sauce

When local tomatoes are in season where you live, make a double or triple batch of this recipe and then freeze it to have on hand during the out-of-season months. Canned tomatoes can be substituted. The sauce is an excellent source of lycopene, and cooking it with olive oil helps with the lycopene absorption.

Serving Suggestions: Spoon over pasta, broiled fish, pizzas, or any dish that calls for a tomato sauce.

MAKES $2\frac{1}{2}$–3 CUPS.
Prep: 15 minutes / Cook: about 25 minutes

> 1 teaspoon olive oil
>
> 1 medium-size onion, chopped
>
> 2 cloves garlic, finely chopped
>
> 3 pounds tomatoes, peeled, seeded, and chopped, or 1 can (28 ounces) whole tomatoes, chopped, with liquid
>
> 1 teaspoon salt
>
> 1 bay leaf
>
> Pinch dried thyme
>
> $\frac{1}{4}$ teaspoon black pepper

1. In a nonstick medium-size saucepan, heat oil over medium heat. Add onion and cook, stirring frequently, until softened, about 5 minutes. Add garlic and cook, stirring frequently, another 2 minutes.

2. Add tomatoes, salt, bay leaf, and thyme. Bring to a boil. Reduce heat slightly and gently boil, stirring occasionally, until thickened, 15 to 20 minutes. Discard bay leaf and stir in pepper.

Make-Ahead Tip: Sauce can be refrigerated for up to three days or frozen for up to six months.

Homemade All-Purpose Tomato Sauce

Here is a basic sauce for pasta dishes, hero sandwiches (page 74), pizza (pages 226–229), and any other recipe that calls for tomato sauce. Because the sauce relies on canned tomatoes and tomato paste, you can make it any time of year, regardless of the availability of flavorful ripe tomatoes. And, since there is no seasoning other than salt, you can jazz it up according to your own taste: basil, oregano, thyme, rosemary, marjoram, in any combination (see Add-Ins that follow).

The canned tomatoes and the tomato paste are excellent sources of lycopene, and the olive oil used for the cooking enhances the lycopene absorption. There are some very good brands of commercially prepared organic meatless marinara sauces that you can use when time is really short—sample them and decide which ones are your favorites.

MAKES ABOUT $3\frac{1}{2}$ CUPS SAUCE
Prep: 10 minutes / Cook: 55 minutes

> 2 tablespoons olive oil
> $\frac{1}{2}$ small sweet onion such as Vidalia, finely chopped
> 2 carrots, trimmed, peeled, and finely chopped
> 2 celery stalks, finely chopped
> 2 cloves garlic, finely chopped
> 1 can (28 ounces) diced tomatoes in juice, or whole tomatoes in juice, cut up
> $\frac{1}{4}$ cup tomato paste
> $\frac{1}{2}$ teaspoon salt
> $\frac{1}{4}$ teaspoon crushed red pepper flakes (optional)

1. In a medium-size nonstick saucepan, heat oil over medium heat. Add onion and cook, stirring occasionally, until softened, about 5 minutes. Add carrots, celery, and garlic and cook, stirring occasionally, for 1 minute.

2. Stir in tomatoes with their juice, tomato paste, salt, and pepper flakes, if using. Simmer, stirring occasionally, for 30 minutes. Add more seasonings to taste (see below).

3. In a blender or food processor, puree the tomato mixture until almost smooth. Return sauce to the pan (see below) and simmer for 15 minutes longer. (If it becomes too thick, add a couple of spoonfuls of water.)

Make-Ahead Tip: Sauce can be refrigerated for up to three days, or frozen for up to a month.

Add-Ins: You can add any one of the following or a combination. When you add tomatoes to the saucepan in step 2, toss in 2 tablespoons grated Parmesan-style soy cheese, $\frac{1}{2}$ teaspoon crushed fennel seeds, and 2 teaspoons dried basil, marjoram, oregano, or Italian seasoning blend. After blending in step 3, you can stir in: $\frac{1}{4}$ to $\frac{1}{3}$ cup finely chopped sun-dried tomatoes, $\frac{1}{3}$ cup finely chopped fresh basil leaves, $\frac{1}{4}$ cup finely chopped fresh parsley leaves, $\frac{1}{2}$ cup finely chopped pitted black or green olives, or 2 tablespoons drained capers, or any combination of the above. Continue cooking as directed.

Tomato-Garlic Sauce with Paprika

The paprika gives the sauce a little edge, especially if you use a spicy version. You can also jazz up the sauce a little more with your favorite herbs and spices, such as basil, tarragon, marjoram, thyme, rosemary, cumin, cinnamon, or curry. The tomatoes are a good source of lycopene. Figure on about a minimum $\frac{1}{2}$ cup of sauce for four servings of vegetables.

Serving Suggestions: Toss with any vegetable you like, fresh or frozen.

MAKES 1 CUP
Prep: 10 minutes / Cook: 5 minutes

> 1 can (14.5 ounces) diced tomatoes
>
> 1 teaspoon olive oil
>
> 2 cloves garlic, finely chopped
>
> 1 teaspoon Hungarian paprika
>
> $\frac{1}{4}$ teaspoon salt
>
> $\frac{1}{8}$ teaspoon black pepper

In a small nonstick saucepan, combine all the ingredients. Bring to a boil. Lower heat and simmer vigorously, stirring occasionally, until the sauce thickens, about 5 minutes. Toss with vegetables.

Make-Ahead Tip: Sauce can be refrigerated for up to three days, then gently reheated in a small nonstick saucepan to serve.

Roasted Garlic Sauce

As the whole head of garlic roasts in the oven, the pulp softens and takes on a rich, sweet flavor. For an Asian flavor boost, add 1 teaspoon peeled, finely chopped fresh ginger to the saucepan when heating the sauce. The added bonus in this recipe is the leftover roasted garlic, which can work its way into many different dishes, as described below.

Serving Suggestions: The sauce can be tossed with most vegetables: broccoli florets, string beans, snow peas, sugar snap peas, cauliflower florets, or zucchini slices, to mention just a few. Use the extra roasted garlic for a delicious meal accompaniment or a snack—scoop out the warm cloves from their skin and spread on crusty bread or crostini (page 56), stir into hot soups, or spread on sandwiches.

MAKES ABOUT $\frac{1}{4}$ CUP SAUCE
Prep: 5 minutes / Cook: 1 hour

1 whole head garlic

1 tablespoon olive oil

$\frac{1}{4}$ cup vegetable broth, homemade (page 101) or store-bought

1. Heat oven to 350°F.

2. Cut about $\frac{1}{2}$ inch off the top of the head of garlic. Remove loose papery outer skin from head. Place head on piece of aluminum foil and drizzle oil over the top. Wrap the garlic up in foil.

3. Roast until garlic is soft, about 1 hour. Check by unwrapping the head of garlic and carefully squeezing it, or slip a knife into a clove to check softness. Remove garlic from the oven and let cool slightly.

4. In a small nonstick saucepan, heat broth. Squeeze enough pulp from individual cloves to make about 1 tablespoon into broth. Stir. Heat through, stirring to evenly distribute garlic throughout sauce.

Make-Ahead Tip: Sauce can be refrigerated for up to three days. Gently reheat it in a small nonstick saucepan. Remaining roasted garlic pulp can be refrigerated in small glass jar for up to three days. Gently reheat it with a little olive oil in a small nonstick skillet or saucepan over low heat, stirring constantly to prevent scorching.

Yogurt-Scallion Sauce

A nice accent spooned over steamed vegetables or served with fish.

MAKES ABOUT $\frac{1}{2}$ CUP
Prep: 5 minutes

$\frac{1}{2}$ cup plain soy yogurt

2 tablespoons finely chopped scallion (2 scallions)

1 teaspoon Dijon mustard

1 teaspoon freshly squeezed lemon juice

Pinch salt

Pinch black pepper

In a small bowl, stir together all the ingredients.

Make-Ahead Tip: Sauce can be refrigerated for up to three days—the flavor of the scallions will become more pronounced.

Spicy Asian Lime Sauce

If you love food from Southeast Asia, then this sauce will hit the mark. The flavors are very strong, but as is often the case in Thai or Vietnamese cooking, they are delicately balanced between salty, sweet, sour, and spicy. Asian fish sauces—the Thai *nam pla* and Vietnamese *nuoc mam*—can be found in the international food sections of most supermarkets or at Asian grocery stores.

Serving Suggestions: Use sparingly. Toss with cooked string beans, sliced carrots, broccoli florets, and any other vegetable you like. Try as a salad dressing or drizzle over sliced tomatoes. Also delicious spooned over a strongly flavored fish such as bluefish or salmon, before broiling, grilling, or roasting. Drizzle a little more over the cooked fish just before serving.

MAKES ABOUT 1 CUP
Prep: 10 minutes

6 tablespoons freshly squeezed lime juice (2–3 limes)

3 tablespoons Asian fish sauce (Thai *nam pla* or Vietnamese *nuoc mam*)

2 tablespoons organic sugar (evaporated cane juice)

3 tablespoons warm water

1 clove garlic, finely chopped

1–2 fresh serrano chiles, cored, seeded, and finely chopped

In a small bowl or glass jar with a tight-fitting lid, combine all the ingredients until sugar is dissolved.

Make-Ahead Tip: Sauce can be refrigerated in a glass jar for up to a week.

Chipotle Mayonnaise

The honey in this mayonnaise balances the fire of the chipotle chiles. This is so good on so many things. Chipotle chiles are smoked and dried jalapeño chiles and can be found canned in a spicy adobo sauce, in the Mexican or Hispanic food section of your supermarket. The calories and fat in this recipe are about the same as you would find in a commercially prepared reduced-fat mayonnaise. The difference is that by starting with a soy-based mayo, there are no eggs and no animal fat.

Serving Suggestions: Substitute this spicy sandwich spread for regular mayonnaise in your favorite tuna fish salad recipe or enliven simple sandwiches, such as sliced tomato and bottled roasted red pepper on toasted whole-grain bread. Spread over the top of a fish fillet such as cod, haddock, or bluefish, and then broil.

MAKES 1 CUP
Prep: 5 minutes

> 2 canned chipotle chiles in adobo
> 1 teaspoon adobo sauce from can
> 1 cup eggless soy-based mayonnaise
> $\frac{1}{8}$ teaspoon salt
> 1 teaspoon honey, or to taste

1. In a blender or small food processor, puree chiles with adobo sauce.

2. In a small bowl, stir together mayonnaise, pureed chiles, salt, and honey.

Make-Ahead Tip: Mayonnaise can be refrigerated for up to a week.

Gremolata

Gremolata is a perky-tasting mixture of chopped garlic, lemon zest, and parsley that is traditionally used in Italian cooking to add a fresh note to stews, but it can be sprinkled into any dish where you want a citrus-garlic accent. A tablespoon or two is usually enough for four servings—experiment to see how much you like.

Serving Suggestions: Toss with green beans, snow peas, broccoli, sauteed kale, or steamed spinach, or sprinkle over leafy green salads or vegetable salads, or pasta and vegetarian stews and soups.

MAKES ABOUT $\frac{1}{4}$ CUP
Prep: 10 minutes

$\frac{1}{4}$ cup chopped fresh flat-leaf parsley

2 cloves garlic, finely chopped

Grated zest of 1 lemon

In a small bowl, stir together all the ingredients.

Make-Ahead Tip: Gremolata can be prepared a day ahead and refrigerated.

BREAKFAST, BRUNCH & 'TEA BREAK

BREAKFAST IS AN IMPORTANT MEAL SINCE it sets the tone for the rest of the day, providing protein and energy after a night of sleep and fasting. I often take an early morning run, looking forward to breakfast when I return home. (It goes without saying that exercise is important in the prevention of disease as well as in the management of prostate cancer.)

My breakfast is always sparse, always low in fat, always high in fiber, and with a little protein. It usually includes a fruit salad for antioxidants, fiber, vitamins, and a natural energy boost. A favorite combination is watermelon, papaya (both good sources of lycopene), and strawberries, topped with cubed firm tofu for protein.

If you're used to a bacon-and-eggs type of breakfast and have the time to fix it, then there are alternatives, such as Baked Chile Grits with Cheese (page 268), Tofu Scramble with Mushrooms and Thyme (page 271), that looks and tastes like the egg version, and Sweet Potato Skillet Hash with Red Bell Pepper (page 270). All of these have only 1 gram of saturated fat and no cholesterol. Are you a pancake lover? There are pumpkin (page 275) and blueberry (page 274) pancakes, both made with unsweetened soy milk and a mixture of whole-wheat pastry flour and all-purpose flour, and rich with antioxidants.

If time is really short, then a blended fruit drink or smoothie, full of flavor as well as antioxidants and fiber, should easily fit into the schedule. Turn to Chapter II, Snacks & Drinks (page 40) for those recipes. It's worth investing in an immersible drink blender to keep the preparation easy.

A downfall for a lot of people are the fat- and calorie-laden muffins that are huge enough to feed four. A low-fat alternative, but still extremely tasty, is a Banana Spice Muffin (page 282)—less than 100 calories, with only 7 grams of (mostly polyunsaturated and monosaturated) fat and 4 grams of fiber. Or try Lemon Poppy Seed Bread with Lemon Glaze (page 276) and Whole-Grain Soda Bread with Cranberries (page 278). These travel well, too.

Whatever your choice for breakfast, remember portion control and keep it low-calorie, low-fat, and high-fiber.

Baked Chile Grits with Cheese

This easy breakfast dish, which also makes a great lunch or light supper, lends itself to endless variations. Use the recipe as a starting point and experiment with your own favorite additions, such as sliced mushrooms, chopped red bell pepper, frozen peas, frozen edamame, frozen chopped collard greens or spinach, and on and on. And take note: in the ingredient list there are a couple of ways you can add heat. Or you can omit the heat altogether. Leftovers are delicious as a snack directly from the refrigerator.

Serving Suggestions: Accompany with a fruit salad or, for lunch, a spinach and tomato salad.

MAKES 6 SERVINGS
Prep: 10 minutes / Cook: 55 minutes

2 tablespoons light olive oil, plus additional for coating baking dish

1 cup chopped scallions (about 1 bunch)

2 cloves garlic, finely chopped

$\frac{1}{4}$ cup pickled jalapeños, chopped, or 1 fresh jalapeño or serrano chile, cored, seeded, and chopped, or 1–2 canned chipotle chiles in adobo, seeded and chopped

2 teaspoons chili powder

2 cups vegetable broth, homemade (page 101) or store-bought

1 cup old-fashioned grits (not quick-cooking)

$\frac{1}{2}$ cup liquid egg substitute

1 cup frozen corn kernels, thawed

1 cup (4 ounces) shredded cheddar-style soy cheese

$\frac{1}{4}$ teaspoon salt

1. Heat oven to 375°F. Lightly coat a 9-inch pie plate with oil.

2. In a medium-size nonstick saucepan, heat oil over medium heat. Add scallions and cook, stirring occasionally, until softened, about 3 minutes. Add garlic, jalapeños, and chili powder and cook, stirring, for 1 minute. Add broth and bring to a boil. Reduce heat to low and gradually whisk in grits. Cook, stirring constantly, until grits thicken, about 2 minutes. Remove from heat.

3. In a small bowl, whisk egg substitute. Quickly whisk a small amount of hot grits into egg substitute. Stir into grits in saucepan. Stir in corn, cheese, and salt. Pour into the prepared pie plate.

4. Bake, uncovered, until golden, about 45 minutes. Let stand for 5 minutes before serving.

Make-Ahead Tip: Grits can be refrigerated for up to two days. Reheat in a 350°F oven or in a microwave. Or snack on small portions that are at room temperature or chilled.

Sweet Potato Skillet Hash with Red Bell Pepper

The sweet potato and red bell pepper provide antioxidants, and the meatless bacon creates the taste of meat without adding the saturated fat.

Serving Suggestions: Arrange slices of cantaloupe, watermelon, and papaya on plates for a fruit salad.

MAKES 4 SERVINGS

Prep: 10 minutes / Cook: about 35 minutes

Nonstick olive oil cooking spray

$1\frac{1}{2}$ pounds sweet potatoes or Yukon Gold potatoes, peeled (or leave skins on) and diced

3 teaspoons olive oil

1 sweet onion such as Vidalia, chopped

1 small red bell pepper, seeded and chopped

4 slices nonmeat soy bacon, cut into small pieces, or 2 ounces meatless breakfast sausages, cut into small pieces

$\frac{1}{2}$ teaspoon dried rosemary, crushed

$\frac{1}{4}$ teaspoon salt

$\frac{1}{4}$ teaspoon black pepper

1. Heat oven to 375°F. Lightly coat a baking sheet with cooking spray. In a medium-size bowl, toss together potatoes with 1 teaspoon of the oil. Spread potatoes in even layer on the sheet.

2. Bake potatoes until tender and lightly colored, 20 to 25 minutes.

3. About 10 minutes before potatoes are done, in a large nonstick skillet, heat the remaining oil over medium heat. Add onion and cook, stirring occasionally, until slightly softened, about 4 minutes. Add bell pepper and cook until pepper and onion are softened, about 3 minutes. Add cooked potatoes, bacon or sausage, rosemary, salt, and pepper and cook, stirring occasionally, until hash is lightly browned and heated through, about 5 minutes. Serve immediately.

Make-Ahead Tip: Hash can be made a day ahead and refrigerated. Reheat it in a skillet with a little olive oil. Cooked hash can be frozen for up to a month, thawed in a microwave, and reheated in a skillet with a little oil or in a microwave.

Tofu Scramble with Mushrooms and Thyme

By using a combination of spices and silken or soft tofu, you actually think you're eating scrambled eggs, and turmeric (thought by some to have prostate-cancer fighting properties, page 38) contributes to the effect by coloring the tofu a scrambled-egg yellow. You can substitute 1 to 2 cups of leftover cooked vegetables—broccoli, bell peppers, or corn—for the mushrooms.

Gauging the percentage of calories from fat in a recipe can be misleading with regard to overall health benefits. This recipe is a good example of that. Since the calories are low, 113, and the fat calculates at 7 grams per serving, the percentage of overall fat is high. But there is still only 1 gram of saturated fat per serving, there is no cholesterol, and the soy provides nonanimal protein and isoflavones.

Serving Suggestions: Accompany with cherry tomatoes, nonmeat soy bacon, and whole-wheat English muffins, or Whole-Grain Soda Bread with Cranberries (page 278).

MAKES 4 SERVINGS
Prep: 5 minutes / Cook: about 12 minutes.

    1 pound silken or soft tofu
    1 tablespoon light olive oil, or a little more as needed
    3 scallions, trimmed and finely chopped
    6–8 ounces mushrooms such as portobello, cremini, or white button, cleaned, tough
      stems removed, and mushrooms sliced
    $\frac{1}{4}$ cup chopped bottled roasted red pepper, blotted dry with paper towels
    $\frac{1}{2}$ teaspoon ground turmeric
    $\frac{1}{2}$ teaspoon dried thyme
    $\frac{1}{2}$ teaspoon salt
    $\frac{1}{4}$ teaspoon black pepper

1. Scoop tofu into a colander, breaking it up into small pieces. Let excess water drain off.

2. Meanwhile, in a medium-size skillet, heat oil over medium-high heat. Add scallions and mushrooms and cook, stirring frequently, until mushrooms are browned and release their moisture, about 5 minutes.

3. Add tofu to the skillet. Stir in red pepper, turmeric, thyme, salt, and pepper. Cook, stirring frequently, until tofu releases most of its moisture and mixture resembles scrambled eggs, about 5 minutes.

Nutty Maple French Toast

The background flavor of toasted nuts is what makes this French toast special—and you would never know there's tofu in the batter. The Brazil nuts are perhaps one of the best sources of selenium, and the tofu offers isoflavones.

Serving Suggestions: Top with toasted chopped Brazil nuts or blueberries or cut-up fresh strawberries.

MAKES 4 SERVINGS

Prep: 15 minutes / Cook: about 12 minutes

$\frac{1}{2}$ cup sliced, blanched almonds

$\frac{1}{4}$ cup Brazil nuts

$1\frac{1}{4}$ cups unsweetened soy milk

4 ounces silken tofu, drained and blotted dry with paper towels

1 teaspoon pure vanilla extract

$\frac{1}{4}$ cup maple syrup

$\frac{1}{8}$ teaspoon ground nutmeg

Nonstick olive oil cooking spray

8 slices whole-grain bread

1. In a large, dry nonstick skillet, toast almonds, stirring frequently, over medium heat until lightly colored, 2 to 4 minutes. Remove to a plate. Repeat with Brazil nuts, toasting for about 2 minutes.

2. In a blender or small food processor, grind nuts into a powder. Add soy milk, tofu, vanilla, syrup, and nutmeg and blend until smooth. Pour into a large bowl.

3. Heat oven to 200°F.

4. Lightly coat a skillet with cooking spray. Heat over medium-high heat. Working in batches, dip bread slices in milk mixture and place in the skillet. Cook until browned on both sides, about 5 minutes total. Transfer slices to a baking sheet and keep warm in the oven. Coat the skillet as needed with additional cooking spray.

Make-Ahead Tip: Batter can be refrigerated for up to two days.

Breakfast Burrito with Red Bell Pepper and Zucchini

Firm tofu replaces the eggs in this breakfast burrito, resulting in a healthy amount of soy protein with no cholesterol and very little saturated fat. If you make the tofu mixture ahead and have it on hand in the refrigerator, you can whip up one of these anytime, for lunch, a light dinner, or a snack.

Serving Suggestions: For a fun brunch, serve with Tropical Fruit Salad with Avocado (page 119), Jazzed-Up Canned Black Beans (page 255), or a fruit salad of your own invention.

MAKES 4 SERVINGS

Prep: 15 minutes / Cook: about 12 minutes

> Four 8-inch low-fat flavored flour tortillas
>
> 1 tablespoon olive oil
>
> 1 small red bell pepper, cored, seeded, and chopped
>
> 1 small zucchini, trimmed and chopped
>
> 3 scallions, trimmed and chopped
>
> 14 ounces firm tofu, drained, blottted dry with paper towels and chopped
>
> 2 teaspoons ground cumin
>
> $\frac{1}{4}$ teaspoon salt
>
> $\frac{1}{8}$ teaspoon black pepper
>
> 1 cup bottled salsa

1. Heat oven to 350°F. Stack tortillas and wrap loosely in aluminum foil. Place in oven and warm for about 10 minutes. Remove from oven and let stand.

2. Meanwhile, in a large nonstick skillet, heat oil over medium heat. Add bell pepper and cook, stirring occasionally, until slightly softened, about 3 minutes. Add zucchini and scallions and cook, stirring occasionally, until softened, about 3 minutes. Stir in tofu, cumin, salt, and pepper, and cook, stirring occasionally, until tofu is heated through and mixture is dry, 3 to 5 minutes (you should have about 3 cups filling).

3. Place warmed tortillas on a work surface. Spoon a quarter of tofu mixture in log shape in center of each tortilla. Top each with $\frac{1}{4}$ cup salsa. Fold two opposite sides of tortilla over ends of filling, then roll up into a burrito. Repeat with remaining tortillas and filling.

Blueberry Pancakes

The star in this recipe is the blueberry, the super antioxidant food. Plus, there's the soy milk and its isoflavones. The whole-wheat pastry flour contributes extra fiber. The bottom line is that, even with all these nutritional advantages, the pancakes taste very good.

Serving Suggestions: Drizzle a little maple syrup over the top and accompany with thinly sliced rounds of seedless orange sprinkled with toasted, chopped Brazil nuts.

MAKES ABOUT 10 PANCAKES

Prep: 10 minutes / Cook: about 4 minutes per batch

> 1 cup unbleached all-purpose flour
> $\frac{1}{2}$ cup whole-wheat pastry flour
> 2 teaspoons baking powder
> $\frac{1}{2}$ teaspoon salt
> $1\frac{1}{4}$ cups unsweetened soy milk
> 2 tablespoons honey
> 1 tablespoon light olive oil
> Liquid egg substitute equal to 1 egg
> 1 tablespoon grated lemon zest
> 1 cup blueberries, thawed if frozen and blotted dry with paper towels
> Nonstick olive oil cooking spray

1. In a large bowl, stir together flours, baking powder, and salt.

2. In a small bowl, stir together $\frac{1}{4}$ cup of the soy milk and the honey until honey is dissolved. Stir in remaining soy milk, the olive oil, egg substitute, and zest.

3. Stir soy milk mixture into flour mixture just until blended—do not overmix.

4. Heat oven to 200°F. Lightly coat a large nonstick skillet with cooking spray. Heat the skillet over medium heat.

5. For each pancake, ladle $\frac{1}{3}$ cup batter into the skillet and scatter about 2 tablespoons berries over top. Cook until bubbles appear on top of pancakes, about 2 minutes. Flip pancakes over and cook until bottoms are lightly browned, 1 to 2 minutes. Transfer pancakes to a baking sheet and keep warm in the oven while making remaining pancakes.

Make-Ahead Tip: Leftover pancakes can be frozen in plastic freezer bags for up to a month. Reheat frozen pancakes in a pop-up toaster or toaster oven at 300°F, or in a microwave.

Pumpkin Pancakes

Pumpkin is high in fiber and an excellent source of the antioxidant beta-carotene. The soy milk contributes isoflavones, among other things, and the whole-wheat pastry flour boosts the fiber.

Serving Suggestions: Drizzle a little maple syrup over the top and accompany with a fruit salad made with watermelon, strawberries, and papaya.

MAKES ABOUT 10 PANCAKES
Prep: 10 minutes / Cook: about 4 minutes per batch

> 1 cup unbleached all-purpose flour
> $\frac{1}{2}$ cup whole-wheat pastry flour
> 2 teaspoons baking powder
> $\frac{1}{2}$ teaspoon salt
> $1\frac{1}{4}$ cups unsweetened soy milk
> 2 tablespoons maple syrup
> 1 tablespoon light olive oil
> Liquid egg substitute equal to 1 egg
> $\frac{1}{3}$ cup pumpkin puree (fresh, canned solid-pack, or thawed frozen)
> 1 tablespoon grated orange zest
> Nonstick olive oil cooking spray

1. In a large bowl, stir together flours, baking powder, and salt.

2. In a small bowl, stir together $\frac{1}{4}$ cup of the soy milk and the maple syrup until syrup is dissolved. Stir in remaining soy milk, the olive oil, egg substitute, pumpkin puree, and orange zest.

3. Stir soy milk mixture into flour mixture just until blended, being careful not to overmix.

4. Heat oven to 200°F. Lightly coat a large nonstick skillet with cooking spray. Heat the skillet over medium heat.

5. For each pancake, ladle $\frac{1}{3}$ cup batter into the skillet. Cook until bubbles appear on top of pancakes, about 2 minutes. Flip pancakes over and cook until bottoms are lightly browned, 1 to 2 minutes. Transfer pancakes to a baking sheet and keep warm in the oven while making remaining pancakes.

Make-Ahead Tip: Leftover pancakes can be frozen in plastic freezer bags for up to a month. Reheat frozen pancakes in a pop-up toaster or toaster oven at 300°F, or in a microwave.

Lemon Poppy Seed Bread with Lemon Glaze

Always moist because of the glaze, this quick bread delivers soy isoflavones with the addition of tofu to the batter, and there's 2 grams of fiber per slice.

Serving Suggestions: A thin slice satisfies as a light after-dinner sweet, as a midafternoon snack, or even as a light breakfast with a fruit salad.

MAKES ABOUT 12 SLICES
Prep: 20 minutes / Bake: 50 minutes / Stand: overnight

$\frac{3}{4}$ cup unsweetened soy milk

3 tablespoons poppy seeds

2 tablespoons light olive oil, plus additional for baking pan

1 cup unbleached all-purpose flour, plus additional for baking pan

$\frac{3}{4}$ cup whole-wheat pastry flour

$\frac{3}{4}$ cup organic sugar (evaporated cane juice)

$1\frac{1}{2}$ teaspoons baking powder

$\frac{1}{2}$ teaspoon baking soda

$\frac{1}{4}$ teaspoon salt

$\frac{1}{2}$ cup (4 ounces) firm tofu, drained and blotted dry with paper towels

1 teaspoon pure vanilla extract

$\frac{3}{4}$ teaspoon lemon extract

2 teaspoons grated lemon zest

2 large egg whites

Lemon Glaze (page 313)

1. In a microwave-safe liquid measure or bowl, combine soy milk and poppy seeds. Microwave at full power for 60 to 90 seconds, or until milk just begins to bubble around edges. (This can also be done in a small saucepan over medium heat.) Set aside to steep for 15 minutes.

2. Meanwhile, heat oven to 350°F. Coat a 9 x 5 x 3-inch loaf pan with oil, then lightly dust with flour to coat, tapping out any excess.

3. In a large bowl, whisk together flours, sugar, baking powder, baking soda, and salt. Make a well in the center.

4. In a blender, process poppy seed mixture until seeds are ground, about 1 minute. Add tofu, the 2 tablespoons oil, vanilla, lemon extract, and zest, and blend until smooth. Add egg whites and blend just until combined.

5. Add tofu-poppy seed mixture to well in flour mixture. Stir together just until combined and dry ingredients are evenly moistened. Scrape into the prepared pan and spread level.

6. Bake until a wooden pick inserted in the center comes out clean, 45 to 50 minutes. Place the pan on a wire rack and pierce the loaf in several places, using a long skewer.

7. Gradually spoon lemon glaze over hot bread, adding more as it is absorbed. Let stand to cool completely. For best flavor, wrap airtight and let stand overnight.

Make-Ahead Tip: Bread can be made up to three days ahead, wrapped in plastic and stored in a cool place, or frozen for up to a month.

Whole-Grain Soda Bread with Cranberries

The inspiration for this recipe is the classic Irish soda bread. Tofu and light olive oil replace the shortening or butter that is often used, so there is no saturated fat.

Serving Suggestions: Serve for breakfast or as an afternoon snack, plain or spread with all-fruit raspberry or blueberry jam, or drizzle with honey. Thin wedges are also good toasted.

MAKES 16 WEDGES

Prep: 15 minutes / Bake: 35 minutes

2 tablespoons light olive oil, plus additional for baking sheet

1 cup unbleached all-purpose flour, plus extra for dusting bread

1 cup whole-wheat pastry flour

1 teaspoon baking powder

$\frac{1}{2}$ teaspoon baking soda

$\frac{1}{2}$ teaspoon salt

$\frac{1}{3}$ cup dried cranberries or golden raisins

$\frac{1}{2}$ cup (4 ounces) firm tofu, drained and blotted dry with paper towels

$\frac{1}{3}$ cup unsweetened soy milk, or water

2 tablespoons honey

1 teaspoon grated orange zest

2 teaspoons orange juice

$\frac{1}{2}$ teaspoon caraway seeds (optional)

1. Heat oven to 375°F. Brush a baking sheet with oil.

2. In a large bowl, stir together flours, baking powder, baking soda, salt, and cranberries. Make a well in the center.

3. In a blender or small food processor, blend together tofu, soy milk, the 2 tablespoons oil, honey, orange zest and juice, and caraway seeds, if using, until smooth. Add to well in dry ingredients and stir until just combined and dry ingredients are evenly moistened. Turn out onto a floured board and knead a few times. Shape dough into a ball, pat it into a 6-inch round, and place it on the prepared baking sheet. Score a 4-inch cross on top of the round and lightly dust the top with unbleached flour.

4. Bake until golden brown and hollow-sounding when tapped, about 35 minutes. Transfer bread to a wire rack and let cool completely. To serve, cut into wedges.

Make-Ahead Tip: Bread can be stored at room temperature for up to three days or frozen for a month.

Cranberry-Nut Bread

Whole-wheat pastry flour replaces some of the usual white flour for additional fiber and nutrients, and tofu and light olive oil take the place of the usual saturated fat.

Serving Suggestions: Try this bread for breakfast or as an afternoon snack with green tea.

MAKES 12 SLICES

Prep: 20 minutes / Bake: 50 minutes

2 tablespoons light olive oil, plus additional for baking pan

1 cup unbleached all-purpose flour, plus additional for baking pan

$\frac{3}{4}$ cup whole-wheat pastry flour

$\frac{1}{3}$ cup Brazil nuts, or pecans, chopped

$\frac{1}{4}$ cup wheat germ

$2\frac{1}{4}$ teaspoons baking powder

$\frac{1}{4}$ teaspoon baking soda

$\frac{1}{4}$ teaspoon salt

$\frac{3}{4}$ cup fresh or frozen cranberries, coarsely chopped

$\frac{3}{4}$ cup organic apple cider, or apple juice

$\frac{1}{2}$ cup packed light brown sugar

$\frac{1}{2}$ cup (4 ounces) firm tofu, drained and blotted dry with paper towels

$1\frac{1}{2}$ teaspoons pure vanilla extract

3 large egg whites

1. Heat oven to 350°F. Coat a 9 x 5 x 3-inch loaf pan with oil. Lightly dust the pan with flour to coat, tapping out any excess.

2. In a large bowl, whisk together flours, nuts, wheat germ, baking powder, baking soda, and salt. Make a well in the center. Add cranberries to well.

3. In a blender, blend together cider, sugar, tofu, the 2 tablespoons oil, and vanilla until smooth. Add egg whites and blend just until combined. Add tofu mixture to well in dry ingredients. Stir together until just combined and dry ingredients are evenly moistened. Scrape into the prepared pan and spread level.

4. Bake until a wooden pick inserted in the center comes out clean, 45 to 50 minutes. Place the pan on a wire rack and let cool for 10 minutes. Turn bread out onto rack to cool completely.

Make-Ahead Tip: Bread can be stored at room temperature for up to three days or frozen for a month.

Oat and Nut Scones

This Scottish quick bread contains the traditional oats, along with whole-wheat flour that adds a little more nutritive value and a slightly sweet, nutty flavor. The nut is selenium-rich Brazil, the light olive oil contributes richness and monounsaturated fat, and the soy milk, isoflavones.

Serving Suggestions: Spread with all-fruit apricot jam or serve with honey on the side for drizzling. Delicious for breakfast with a cup of tea or coffee and a bowl of fruit salad, or with Tofu Scramble with Mushrooms and Thyme (page 271).

MAKES 8 SCONES

Prep: 20 minutes / Stand: 30 minutes / Cook: 18 minutes

> 3 tablespoons light olive oil, plus additional for baking sheet
>
> 1 cup unbleached all-purpose flour, plus additional for dusting baking sheet and for shaping
>
> $\frac{1}{2}$ cup unsweetened soy milk
>
> $\frac{3}{4}$ cup old-fashioned rolled oats (not quick-cooking)
>
> $\frac{1}{4}$ cup packed light brown sugar
>
> 1 teaspoon pure vanilla extract
>
> 2 large egg whites
>
> $\frac{3}{4}$ cup whole-wheat pastry flour
>
> $\frac{1}{3}$ cup pecans or Brazil nuts, chopped
>
> $2\frac{1}{2}$ teaspoons baking powder
>
> $\frac{1}{2}$ teaspoon ground allspice (optional)
>
> $\frac{1}{2}$ teaspoon salt

1. Coat baking sheet with oil. Generously sprinkle flour in an 8-inch circle in the center of the sheet.

2. Place soy milk in a microwave-safe measure or bowl. Microwave at full power just until milk begins to simmer, 70 to 90 seconds. (Or bring to a simmer in a small saucepan.) Stir in oats and let stand until cool, about 30 minutes. Then stir in sugar, the 3 tablespoons oil, vanilla, and egg whites until blended.

3. In a large bowl, stir together the cup of all-purpose and the whole-wheat flour, nuts, baking powder, allspice, if using, and salt. Make a well in the center. Add oat mixture and stir together just until combined—dough will be sticky.

4. Heat oven to 400°F.

5. Turn the dough out onto a well-floured board and, with floured hands, shape it into a ball. Place ball on the baking sheet on the floured circle and pat into a 7-inch circle, about $\frac{3}{4}$ inch thick.

6. Bake until golden and firm to touch in center, about 18 minutes. Cut into wedges. Serve warm or at room temperature.

Make-Ahead Tip: Scones can be stored airtight at room temperature for up to three days or frozen for up to a month.

Banana Spice Muffins

This muffin recipe is a good example of how you can substitute applesauce or banana for butter or other animal fat when baking—the result is only 7 grams of fat per muffin, and the majority of that is poly- and monounsaturated. The whole-wheat pastry flour keeps the muffins lighter than if you were using regular whole-wheat flour, and the wheat germ adds a little more fiber, for a total of 4 grams per muffin.

Serving Suggestions: Spread with apricot jam, apple butter, or pumpkin butter. These are delicious any time of day.

MAKES 12 MUFFINS
Prep: 10 minutes / Cook: 25 minutes / Stand: 10 minutes

Nonstick olive oil cooking spray
2 cups whole-wheat pastry flour
2 tablespoons wheat germ
2 teaspoons baking powder
1 teaspoon baking soda
$\frac{1}{2}$ teaspoon salt
1 teaspoon ground cinnamon
$\frac{1}{4}$ teaspoon ground nutmeg
$\frac{1}{3}$ cup organic sugar (evaporated cane juice)
1 cup unsweetened applesauce
2 tablespoons light olive oil
$\frac{1}{3}$ cup unsweetened soy milk
2 bananas, peeled and chopped
$\frac{1}{2}$ cup Brazil nuts or pecans, chopped

1. Heat oven to 350°F. Lightly coat 12 standard-size muffin cups with cooking spray.

2. In a medium-size bowl, stir together flour, wheat germ, baking powder, baking soda, salt, cinnamon, nutmeg, and sugar. Make a well in the center of ingredients. In a small bowl, stir together applesauce, oil, and soy milk. Pour into the well and stir together to make a stiff batter, adding more milk if needed. Fold in banana and nuts. Divide batter equally among the lined cups, about $\frac{1}{4}$ cup each.

3. Bake until a wooden pick inserted in the center of a muffin comes out clean and tops are golden, 20 to 25 minutes. Transfer the muffin pan to a wire rack and let stand for 10 minutes. Remove muffins to the rack and let cool. Serve warm or at room temperature.

Make-Ahead Tip: Muffins can be stored in an airtight container at room temperature for up to three days, or frozen for up to three months.

CHAPTER XI

DESSERTS

DESSERTS ARE A BRIGHT SPOT at the end of a meal, or even as a midafternoon break—they make us smile. Unfortunately, they often rely on fat for their deliciousness, and that means eggs, butter, heavy cream, ricotta cheese, mascarpone, and lots of other wonderful ingredients. However, for the prostate-attuned diet (and healthy heart), the saturated fat found in eggs and dairy products is a no-no. The trick then becomes how to capture the warm satisfaction of fat on the palate. Here are some easy tricks. Substitute packaged refrigerated egg whites or liquid egg substitute for whole eggs. Replace whole milk with soy milk. For cake and cookie baking, substitute applesauce, mashed banana, or prune puree for butter or other fats. Or substitute tofu and light olive oil, as in Carrot Spice Cookies (page 300) or Orange-Almond Snack Cake (page 294). In addition, replacing part of the white flour in baked desserts with whole-wheat pastry flour adds nutrients and fiber. And using pastry flour rather than regular whole-wheat flour makes for a lighter-textured dessert.

Chocolate is another story. Even though the cocoa butter in chocolate contains fatty acids, one of them, stearic acid, has been shown to impede the growth of prostate cancer cells. This doesn't mean you should consume chocolate day and night. It is high in calories, and that means eating too much will put on the pounds. But a little now and then is not a bad thing. The Very Rich Chocolate Mousse (page 309) with tofu is quick to fix and provides a very intense chocolate hit.

Fruit desserts are an easy way to skirt around fat and introduce more fiber into your diet. Dried Fruit and Pear Compote with Chai Tea (page 307) and Apple and Pear Crisp with Cranberries (page 302) are good examples of how to do it. And if you keep antioxidant-rich Pomegranate-Blueberry Ice (page 306) and Citrusy Green Tea Ice (page 305) in the freezer instead of ice cream, you're on the path to success.

For the easiest dessert, cut up some fruit and top it with a sauce such as Creamy Raspberry (page 314) made with silken tofu or just plain Macerated Strawberries (page 317).

A Rich Carrot Bundt Cake

Typically moist and jam-packed with antioxidants thanks to the pound of carrots it contains, this carrot cake is also dense with golden raisins and with Brazil nuts, a rich source of selenium. There are no eggs in this recipe, and tofu and light olive oil replace the usual butter, resulting in a cake that contains about a third of the expected fat. And remember that the nuts contribute a large portion of this fat, so most of it is monounsaturated.

Serving Suggestions: For a special touch, spread the cake with Orange Cream Cheese Frosting (page 312) or poke holes in the top of the cake while it's still warm and spoon warm Orange Glaze (page 313) over the top.

MAKES 16 SLICES

Prep: 15 minutes / Bake: 55 minutes

$^2\!/_3$ cup light olive oil, plus additional for coating baking pan

2 cups unbleached all-purpose flour, plus additional for dusting pan

1 cup whole-wheat pastry flour

2 teaspoons baking powder

1 teaspoon baking soda

1 teaspoon salt

2 teaspoons ground cinnamon

$^1\!/_2$ teaspoon ground nutmeg

$^1\!/_4$ teaspoon ground cloves

1 pound carrots, trimmed and peeled

6 ounces ($^3\!/_4$ cup) firm tofu, drained and blotted dry with paper towels

2 cups firmly packed light brown sugar

2 teaspoons pure vanilla extract

2 tablespoons orange juice concentrate

1 cup Brazil nuts, chopped

1 cup golden raisins

1. Heat oven to 350°F. Lightly coat a 9-inch (9-cup) Bundt or tube cake pan with oil. Dust pan with unbleached all-purpose flour, tapping out excess.

2. In a large bowl, stir together flours, baking powder, baking soda, salt, cinnamon, nutmeg, and cloves until well blended. Make a well in the center.

3. In a food processor with a grating attachment, or with a hand grater, grate carrots. Add to well in dry ingredients.

4. Put the regular blade into the food processor and combine tofu, sugar, the $\frac{2}{3}$ cup oil, vanilla, and juice concentrate. Process until smooth, about 1 minute. Add to well. Stir wet ingredients into dry—the batter will be very stiff. Stir in nuts and raisins. Scrape batter into the prepared pan, smooth top, and rap pan on a hard surface to settle batter.

5. Bake until a wooden pick inserted in the center of the cake comes out clean, about 55 minutes. Transfer pan to a wire rack and let cool slightly, about 10 minutes. Loosen cake from side of pan with a spatula, if necessary. Turn cake out onto the wire rack and let cool completely.

Make-Ahead Tip: Cake can be stored, wrapped in waxed paper and plastic wrap, at cool room temperature for up to three days or frozen for up to a month.

Hazelnut Sponge Cake

A sponge cake is naturally low in fat because it begins with egg whites and no yolks. This version incorporates hazelnuts (or selenium-rich Brazil nuts) for extra richness, whole-wheat pastry flour, and organic sugar, which is purer than the regular refined—and there's only 2 grams of fat per serving, with just a little more than 150 calories.

Serving Suggestions: Macerated Strawberries (page 317) or a scoop of your favorite soy ice cream will easily dress up a slice of this cake, or lightly spread the top of the cake with Orange Cream Cheese Frosting (page 312).

MAKES 12 SERVINGS
Prep: 25 minutes / Cook: 1 hour

1 cup organic sugar (evaporated cane juice)
$\frac{1}{3}$ cup packed light brown sugar
$\frac{1}{3}$ cup toasted chopped hazelnuts, or Brazil nuts
$\frac{1}{2}$ cup sifted whole-wheat pastry flour
$\frac{1}{2}$ cup unbleached all-purpose flour
$\frac{1}{2}$ teaspoon salt
12 large egg whites ($1\frac{1}{2}$ cups), at room temperature
1 teaspoon cream of tartar, or 2 teaspoons freshly squeezed lemon juice
2 tablespoons hazelnut liqueur (optional)
$1\frac{1}{2}$ teaspoons pure vanilla extract

1. Set the oven rack in the lower third of oven. Heat oven to 325°F.

2. In a food processor or blender, and working in 2 batches if necessary, blend together organic and brown sugars until very finely ground, about 2 minutes. Remove $\frac{3}{4}$ cup of sugar mixture and set aside. Add nuts to food processor and blend, using on-and-off pulses until nuts are chopped medium-fine. Place sugar-nut mixture in a large bowl. Add flours and salt and whisk together until well blended.

3. Place egg whites in the large bowl of an electric mixer. Beat on low speed until frothy, about 2 minutes. Add cream of tartar and beat until soft and fluffy, about 2 minutes more. Increase speed to medium and beat in the reserved $\frac{3}{4}$ cup sugar mixture a tablespoon at a time, until shiny, soft peaks form—do not overbeat. Beat in hazelnut liqueur, if using, and vanilla just until blended.

4. Sprinkle a rounded $\frac{1}{4}$ cup of flour-sugar mixture over egg whites. Using a large rubber spatula, gently fold in flour mixture until almost combined. Repeat with remaining flour mixture, being careful not to overmix. Spoon batter into a 10 x 4-inch straight-sided tube pan and spread level. Rap pan on counter a few times to release any large air bubbles.

5. Bake until top springs back when firmly pressed, 50 to 60 minutes. Invert tube pan onto a bottleneck or inverted metal funnel and let stand until completely cooled, 2 to 3 hours. Loosen cake from pan by running a sharp, thin-bladed knife around edges and center tube. Invert onto a plate or cake rack, remove pan, and then return cake right side up. Slice cake with serrated knife.

Make-Ahead Tip: Cake, wrapped airtight, can be stored at room temperature for up to four days or frozen for up to a month.

Chocolate Pudding Cake

Served warm, this luscious dessert registers at only about 100 calories and 3 grams of fat—hard to believe. The silken tofu adds a creamy texture and thickens the sauce, a task usually accomplished by eggs. Replacing some of the white flour with whole-wheat pastry flour adds nutrients and fiber, while making for a lighter cake than if using regular whole-wheat flour, which contains more protein. There is some speculation that a particular active ingredient in chocolate may inhibit the growth of prostate cancer—but that shouldn't be used as an excuse for eating more than one serving of this at a sitting.

Serving Suggestions: A nondairy vanilla ice cream is the perfect accompaniment (I like It's Soy Delicious brand). If you want to be really wicked, a tiny dollop of sweetened whipped cream is also very tasty.

MAKES 10 SERVINGS

Prep: 15 minutes / Cook: 30 minutes / Stand: 30 minutes

> 1 tablespoon light olive oil, plus additional for pan
>
> $\frac{1}{2}$ cup whole-wheat pastry flour
>
> $\frac{1}{2}$ cup all-purpose flour
>
> 2 teaspoons baking powder
>
> $\frac{1}{2}$ teaspoon salt
>
> 1 cup organic sugar (evaporated cane juice)
>
> $\frac{1}{2}$ cup Dutch process or unsweetened cocoa powder
>
> 1 teaspoon pure vanilla extract
>
> $1\frac{3}{4}$ cups very hot water
>
> $\frac{1}{2}$ cup (4 ounces) silken tofu, drained and blotted dry with paper towels
>
> $\frac{1}{2}$ teaspoon espresso or instant coffee powder
>
> Nondairy vanilla ice cream, for serving (optional)

1. Heat oven to 350°F. Brush the bottom and sides of a 9-inch square baking dish with oil.

2. In a medium-size bowl, stir together flours, baking powder, salt, $\frac{2}{3}$ cup of the sugar, and $\frac{1}{4}$ cup of the cocoa powder. Make a well in the center and add $\frac{1}{2}$ cup water, the 1 tablespoon oil, and vanilla. Stir together just until combined and mixture is evenly moistened. Spoon batter into baking pan and spread level.

3. In a blender or small food processor, blend together the $1\frac{3}{4}$ cups very hot water, the tofu, espresso powder, the remaining $\frac{1}{3}$ cup sugar, and $\frac{1}{4}$ cup cocoa powder until smooth. Pour over the back of a spoon into the batter to gently divert liquid over the surface.

4. Bake until slightly firm to touch in the center, about 30 minutes—the top pudding layer will still be very liquidy. Let the dish cool on a wire rack for 30 minutes. Serve warm, with nondairy ice cream, if desired.

Make-Ahead Tip: Dessert can be made a day ahead, refrigerated, and then when ready to serve, gently rewarmed in a microwave at full power for about a minute, or in a 350°F oven for about 3 minutes.

Surprise Chocolate-Layer Cake

Molly, my honorary niece, showed me a very intriguing recipe in one of her children's books when she was six. It was an old Southern favorite, a chocolate cake with tomato in the batter. When I told her it was a good idea for this book (because of the lycopene), she, along with her mother, who is a registered dietician, tested and modified the recipe. Here it is—the olive oil, tomato puree, and egg whites make the cake healthier than it would appear. Cocoa powder contains less fat than regular chocolate (there are only 2 grams per serving in this dessert), and there is no cholesterol because there are no egg yolks or butter.

MAKES 12 SERVINGS
Prep: 20 minutes / Cook: 35 minutes

1 cup light olive oil, plus additional for coating baking pan

$2\frac{1}{2}$ cups unbleached all-purpose flour, plus additional for dusting pan

$1\frac{3}{4}$ cups organic sugar (evaporated cane juice)

$\frac{1}{2}$ cup unsweetened cocoa powder

$1\frac{1}{2}$ teaspoons baking soda

1 teaspoon salt

5 large egg whites

$\frac{1}{2}$ cup canned tomato puree

1 teaspoon pure vanilla extract

$\frac{1}{4}$ cup all-fruit raspberry or strawberry jam

$\frac{1}{4}$ cup confectioners' sugar

1. Heat oven to 350°F. Lightly coat two $8\frac{1}{2}$ x 2-inch round layer-cake pans with oil. Dust pans with flour, tapping out excess.

2. In a large bowl, whisk together flour, sugar, cocoa powder, baking soda, and salt.

3. In a medium-size bowl, stir together 2 of the egg whites, the cup of olive oil, $\frac{3}{4}$ cup cold water, the tomato puree, and vanilla. Stir into flour mixture until blended, but not overmixed.

4. In a clean medium-size bowl, beat the remaining 3 egg whites until stiff but not dry peaks form. Fold into batter. Divide batter equally between the prepared pans.

5. Bake until a wooden pick inserted in the center of the cake comes out clean and sides begin to pull away from the pans, about 35 minutes. Let cakes cool in the pans on wire racks for 10 minutes. Run a thin knife around the side of each pan and turn cakes out onto the racks. Let cool completely.

6. To assemble, spread jam over top of one layer. Stack the second layer on top. Using a small fine-mesh sieve, dust the top with confectioners' sugar.

Make-Ahead Tip: Cake layers, well wrapped, can be stored at room temperature for up to three days or frozen for up to a month. The assembled cake can be refrigerated for up to two days.

Orange-Almond Snack Cake

Delicious for dessert or for snacking—just make the portions smaller for snacking. Light olive oil and silken tofu replace the standard whole eggs and butter. There is no alpha-linolenic acid in almonds, as in other nuts, and this compound is thought to increase the risk of prostate cancer.

Serving Suggestions: Eat as is, dust with confectioners' sugar, or spread with Lemon or Orange Glaze (page 313) or Orange Cream Cheese Frosting (page 312). Or you could always pour on a little Hot Chocolate Sauce (page 316).

MAKES 16 SQUARES
Prep: 20 minutes / Bake: 25 minutes

$\frac{1}{4}$ cup plus 2 tablespoons sliced almonds

3 tablespoons light olive oil, plus additional for coating baking pan

$\frac{2}{3}$ cup unbleached all-purpose flour, plus additional for dusting pan

1 cup whole-wheat pastry flour

$\frac{1}{2}$ teaspoon baking powder

$\frac{1}{2}$ teaspoon baking soda

$\frac{1}{4}$ teaspoon salt

$\frac{1}{2}$ cup (4 ounces) silken tofu, drained and blotted dry with paper towels

$\frac{1}{2}$ cup packed light brown sugar

$\frac{1}{3}$ cup honey

3 tablespoons orange juice concentrate

2 teaspoons grated orange zest

$\frac{1}{4}$ teaspoon almond extract

2 large egg whites

1. Heat oven to 350°F. Place $\frac{1}{4}$ cup of the almonds on a baking sheet and set in preheating oven. Bake until nuts are golden brown, 6 to 8 minutes, stirring occasionally. Transfer nuts to a plate and set aside.

2. Brush the bottom and sides of an 8 x 8 x 2-inch square baking pan with oil. Dust with flour to coat, tapping out excess.

3. In a large bowl, whisk together flours, baking powder, baking soda, and salt. Make a well in the center.

4. In a blender or food processor, process together tofu, sugar, honey, $\frac{1}{4}$ cup water, orange juice concentrate, the 3 tablespoons oil, orange zest, almond extract, and toasted almonds until smooth and almonds are finely ground. Add egg whites and process just until combined. Pour into well in dry ingredients. Stir just until blended and dry ingredients are evenly moistened. Scrape batter into the prepared pan and spread level. Sprinkle the remaining 2 tablespoons sliced almonds evenly on top.

5. Bake until cake springs back when lightly pressed in the center, about 25 minutes. Place pan on a wire rack and let cool for at least 30 minutes. Cut into squares and serve.

Make-Ahead Tip: Cake can be stored, wrapped, at cool room temperature, for up to three days or frozen for up to a month.

Spicy Gingerbread

No whole eggs or the usual saturated fat-laden butter or shortening in this gingerbread. Instead, light olive oil contributes the taste of fat, silken tofu adds richness and moisture, and whole-wheat pastry flour replaces some of the white flour. Fresh ginger is the secret to the hot spiciness.

Serving Suggestions: Dust with confectioners' sugar, or top warm gingerbread with a scoop of nondairy ice cream. For a fancier version, spread cake with Lemon Glaze (page 313) or Orange Cream Cheese Frosting (page 312).

MAKES 12 SLICES
Prep: 20 minutes / Cook: 30 minutes

3 tablespoons light olive oil, plus additional for coating baking pan

$\frac{1}{2}$ cup unbleached all-purpose flour, plus additional for dusting pan

1 cup whole-wheat pastry flour

$\frac{1}{2}$ teaspoon baking powder

$\frac{1}{2}$ teaspoon baking soda

$1\frac{1}{2}$ teaspoons ground cinnamon

$1\frac{1}{2}$ teaspoons ground ginger

$\frac{1}{4}$ teaspoon ground cloves, or nutmeg

$\frac{3}{4}$ teaspoon salt

$\frac{1}{2}$ cup (4 ounces) silken tofu, drained and blotted dry with paper towels

$\frac{1}{2}$ cup dark organic molasses

$\frac{1}{3}$ cup packed light brown sugar

$\frac{1}{4}$ cup unsweetened soy milk

2 teaspoons peeled, grated fresh ginger (see Note below)

2 large egg whites

1. Heat oven to 350°F. Coat a 9 x 1-inch round cake pan with oil, then dust lightly with flour, tapping out excess.

2. In a large bowl, whisk together flours, baking powder, baking soda, cinnamon, ginger, cloves, and salt until combined. Make a well in the center.

3. In a blender or food processor, process together tofu, molasses, sugar, soy milk, the 3 tablespoons oil, and fresh ginger until smooth. Add egg whites and process just until combined. Pour into well in dry ingredients. Stir together just until combined and dry

ingredients are evenly moistened. Scrape batter into the prepared pan and spread level.

4. Bake until cake springs back when lightly pressed in the center, about 30 minutes. Place the pan on a wire rack and let cool for at least 30 minutes. Cut into wedges and serve warm or at room temperature.

Note: A teaspoon of ground ginger can be substituted for the fresh, making a total of $2\frac{1}{2}$ teaspoons ground ginger in the recipe.

Make-Ahead Tip: Gingerbread can be stored, wrapped, at cool room temperature for up to three days or frozen for up to a month.

Mini Cheesecakes with Blueberry Topping

The problem with these soy-based bite-size cheesecakes is that you run the risk of eating all of them at once. Each mini is only about 100 calories with 1 gram of saturated fat—and of course, no cholesterol. The silken tofu duplicates the creaminess of a full-fat cheesecake. You can substitute coarsely chopped strawberries for the blueberries in the topping. The soy cream cheese does contain a small amount of partially hydrogenated oil, though, so save these for a special indulgence.

MAKES 10 MINI CHEESECAKES

Prep: 20 minutes / Bake: 14 minutes / Refrigerate: 1 hour

 Nonstick olive oil cooking spray

 1 cup (8 ounces) silken tofu, drained and blotted dry with paper towels

 $\frac{1}{3}$ cup nondairy imitation cream cheese (soy-based), at room temperature

 $\frac{1}{3}$ cup organic sugar (evaporated cane juice)

 2 tablespoons unbleached all-purpose flour

 $\frac{1}{4}$ cup liquid egg substitute

 2 teaspoons grated lemon zest

 1 tablespoon freshly squeezed lemon juice

 1 teaspoon pure vanilla extract

 3 tablespoons all-fruit seedless raspberry or blueberry jam

 1 cup fresh or frozen blueberries (see Note below)

1. Heat oven to 300°F. Line 10 regular-size muffin pan cups with paper liners and lightly coat bottoms of papers with cooking spray.

2. In a blender or small food processor, blend together tofu, soy cream cheese, sugar, flour, egg substitute, lemon zest and juice, and vanilla until smooth. Spoon batter into paper liners, about 3 scant tablespoons per cup.

3. Bake cheesecakes until slightly puffed and set in centers, about 14 minutes—they may begin to crack and will be moist to the touch. Cool cheesecakes in the pan on a wire rack. Refrigerate until chilled.

4. When cheesecakes have cooled, in a microwave-safe bowl, heat jam in microwave at full power just until jam begins to bubble, about 15 seconds. Stir until smooth. Gently stir in blueberries until evenly coated. (This can also be done in a small saucepan over medium-low heat.) Spoon berries over cheesecakes. When cooled, serve.

Note: If using frozen blueberries, spread out in a single layer on paper towels until thawed, then gently blot dry with paper towels. Use as directed, tossing with the jam right before serving.

Make-Ahead Tip: Cheesecakes, without the topping, can be refrigerated for up to two days.

Carrot Spice Cookies

Using whole-wheat pastry flour rather than regular whole-wheat flour makes for a lighter cookie because the pastry flour contains less protein. Light olive oil and tofu replace the usual eggs, resulting in no cholesterol and only 1 gram of saturated fat per cookie.

MAKES ABOUT $4\frac{1}{2}$ DOZEN COOKIES
Prep: 20 minutes / Cook: 12–14 minutes per batch

Nonstick olive oil cooking spray
1 cup whole-wheat pastry flour
1 cup unbleached all-purpose flour
$1\frac{1}{4}$ teaspoons ground cinnamon
$\frac{3}{4}$ teaspoon ground ginger
$\frac{1}{4}$ teaspoon ground nutmeg
$\frac{1}{2}$ teaspoon baking soda
$\frac{1}{2}$ teaspoon salt
$\frac{1}{3}$ cup chopped Brazil nuts or almonds
$\frac{1}{3}$ cup chopped dates or prunes
1 cup organic sugar (evaporated cane juice)
$\frac{1}{2}$ cup (4 ounces) firm tofu, drained and blotted dry with paper towels
$\frac{1}{4}$ cup plus 2 tablespoons light olive oil
1 teaspoon pure vanilla extract
$\frac{3}{4}$ cup finely shredded carrot (about 2 carrots)

1. Heat oven to 350°F. Lightly coat two baking sheets with cooking spray.

2. In a large bowl, stir together flours, cinnamon, ginger, nutmeg, baking soda, and salt. Stir in nuts and dates. Make a well in the center.

3. In a blender or small food processor, blend together sugar, tofu, oil, and vanilla until smooth. Add to well in dry ingredients. Add carrots to well, and stir just until dry ingredients are evenly moistened.

4. Drop dough by rounded teaspoonfuls onto the prepared baking sheets, spacing cookies $1\frac{1}{2}$ inches apart. Flatten them slightly.

5. Bake until lightly browned around edges, 12 to 14 minutes. Transfer cookies to a wire rack to cool completely.

Make-Ahead Tip: Cookies can be stored in an airtight container at room temperature for up to a week or frozen for up to a month.

Oatmeal Cookies with Cranberries and Brazil Nuts

Olive oil substitutes for butter in these otherwise old-fashioned treats, but no one will be the wiser. You don't need an electric mixture—you can mix the ingredients together by hand. Susan McQuillan developed this recipe, and the doormen in her apartment building voted thumbs-up after they had tasted the samples. And they probably didn't realize that there is 1 gram of fiber per cookie.

MAKES $3\frac{1}{2}$ DOZEN COOKIES
Prep: 10 minutes / Cook 12 minutes per batch

> Nonstick olive oil cooking spray
> 1 cup unbleached all-purpose flour
> $2\frac{1}{2}$ teaspoons baking powder
> $\frac{3}{4}$ teaspoon ground cinnamon
> $\frac{1}{2}$ teaspoon salt
> 1 cup old-fashioned rolled oats (not quick-cooking)
> 2 large egg whites
> $\frac{1}{2}$ cup light olive oil
> 1 teaspoon pure vanilla extract
> 1 cup lightly packed light brown sugar
> $\frac{3}{4}$ cup dried cranberries
> $\frac{3}{4}$ cup Brazil nuts or pecans, finely chopped

1. Heat oven to 375°F. Lightly coat two baking sheets with nonstick cooking spray.

2. In a medium-size bowl, stir together flour, baking powder, cinnamon, and salt. Stir in oats and set aside.

3. In a second medium-size bowl, beat together egg whites, oil, and vanilla. Beat in sugar until well blended. Add flour mixture and stir just until dry ingredients are evenly moistened. Stir in cranberries and nuts.

4. Drop dough by heaping teaspoonfuls onto the prepared baking sheets, spacing them about 2 inches apart.

5. Bake until the tops are lightly golden and the bottoms are browned, about 12 minutes. Transfer the baking sheet to a wire rack and let stand for 2 minutes before transferring cookies to wire racks to cool completely.

Make-Ahead Tip: Cookies can be stored in an airtight container at room temperature for up to a week or frozen for up to a month.

Apple and Pear Crisp with Cranberries

The crumble topping can be used with any combination of fruit, such as peaches and blueberries or pears and dried apricots. Whole-wheat pastry flour replaces the usual white flour in the standard oat topping.

Serving Suggestions: Top with soy yogurt or Creamy Raspberry Sauce (page 314).

MAKES 8 SERVINGS

Prep: 20 minutes / Cook: 35 minutes

- 2 Golden Delicious apples (about 1 pound), with skins on, cored, and sliced about $1/8$ inch thick
- 3 firm, ripe Bartlett pears (about $1\frac{1}{2}$ pounds), with skins on, cored, and sliced about $1/8$ inch thick
- 1 cup fresh or frozen cranberries
- 1 tablespoon cornstarch
- 1 tablespoon freshly squeezed lemon juice
- $1\frac{1}{2}$ teaspoons peeled, grated fresh ginger
- $3/4$ cup packed light brown sugar
- $1\frac{1}{2}$ teaspoons ground cinnamon
- 2 tablespoons light olive oil
- 2 tablespoons honey
- $3/4$ cup whole-wheat pastry flour
- $1/2$ cup old-fashioned rolled or quick oats
- $1/8$ teaspoon salt

1. Heat oven to 375°F.

2. In a large bowl, toss together apples, pears, cranberries, cornstarch, lemon juice, ginger, $1/2$ cup of the sugar, and $1/2$ teaspoon of the cinnamon. Spoon into a shallow 2-quart baking dish, pat down fruit mixture, and spread level.

3. Wipe out the bowl and pour in oil, honey, and remaining $1/4$ cup sugar and stir until blended. Add flour, oats, salt, and the remaining 1 teaspoon cinnamon, and stir until mixture is well combined and crumbly. Sprinkle evenly over the fruit in the baking dish.

4. Bake until fruit is bubbly and topping is golden brown, 30 to 35 minutes. Serve warm or at room temperature.

Make-Ahead Tip: Crisp can be refrigerated for three days. Warm in 350°F oven or microwave.

Strawberry Tiramisu

This is as rich tasting as the popular Italian original, but without the dairy or saturated fat—silken tofu creates the creamy texture. There are several brands of soy cream cheese, but I prefer Tofutti.

MAKES 12 SERVINGS
Prep: 25 minutes / Refrigerate: 6 hours–overnight.

> 4 ounces low-fat or regular ladyfingers (14–20 cookies, 3 or 4 inches long by 1 inch wide), split
>
> 1 pound strawberries, hulled
>
> 3 tablespoons honey
>
> 2 tablespoons orange-flavored liqueur such as Cointreau or Triple Sec
>
> $\frac{1}{2}$ cup unsweetened soy milk
>
> $1\frac{1}{4}$ teaspoons ($\frac{1}{2}$ package) unflavored gelatin
>
> $\frac{3}{4}$ cup (6 ounces) silken tofu, drained and blotted dry with paper towels
>
> $\frac{1}{2}$ cup (4 ounces) nondairy imitation cream cheese (soy-based)
>
> $\frac{1}{3}$ cup packed light brown sugar
>
> $1\frac{1}{2}$ teaspoons grated lemon zest
>
> 2 teaspoons pure vanilla extract

1. Arrange half of the ladyfingers in the bottom of a 9 x 4 x 3-inch loaf pan. Slice half of the strawberries and set aside. In a blender or food processor, combine the remaining berries, honey, and liqueur. Process until pureed. Scrape into a bowl. Do not clean the blender.

2. Pour $\frac{1}{4}$ cup of the soy milk into a microwave-safe liquid measure. Sprinkle gelatin over the top and let stand for 3 minutes to soften. Microwave at full power for 40 to 50 seconds. Stir mixture until gelatin is dissolved. If needed, continue to microwave at 10-second intervals, stirring until dissolved. (This can also be done in a small saucepan over low heat.)

3. In a blender or food processor, combine tofu, cream cheese, sugar, lemon zest, vanilla, the remaining $\frac{1}{4}$ cup soy milk, and gelatin mixture. Blend until smooth, about 30 seconds.

4. Drizzle half of the pureed berries over ladyfingers. Arrange half of the sliced strawberries on top. Spoon half of the tofu mixture over the top, spreading evenly. Repeat layering with the remaining ingredients: ladyfingers, pureed strawberries, sliced strawberries, and tofu mixture. Cover with plastic and refrigerate for at least 6 hours or overnight.

Make-Ahead Tip: Tiramisu can be refrigerated for up to two days.

Soufflé à l'Orange

A little bit of tofu replaces the saturated fat-laden egg yolks in the cooked base. Remember, like all hot soufflés, this needs to be enjoyed straight from the oven. Some may consider this recipe a little finicky, but I think finicky is okay from time to time, if the results are something delicious.

MAKES 4 SERVINGS
Prep: 15 minutes / Cook: 35 minutes

Light olive oil, for soufflé dish

$1\frac{1}{2}$ tablespoons, plus $\frac{1}{3}$ cup, organic sugar (evaporated cane juice)

$\frac{1}{2}$ cup (4 ounces) silken tofu, drained and blotted dry with paper towels

2 teaspoons finely grated orange zest

$\frac{1}{3}$ cup orange juice

3 tablespoons orange-flavored liqueur such as Cointreau or Triple Sec

3 tablespoons unbleached all-purpose flour

1 tablespoon light olive oil

5 large egg whites

1. Heat oven to 350°F. Brush a 6-cup soufflé dish with oil. Sprinkle $1\frac{1}{2}$ tablespoons of the sugar into the dish, turning it to coat sides and bottom.

2. In a blender or small food processor, process together tofu, orange zest and juice, liqueur, flour, and oil until smooth. Pour into a small saucepan. Place on medium heat and cook, whisking constantly, until mixture comes to a simmer, about 3 minutes. Cook for 1 minute more, whisking constantly. Remove from heat.

3. In a large bowl, using an electric mixer, beat egg whites until soft peaks form. Gradually add the remaining $\frac{1}{3}$ cup sugar and beat until stiff but not dry peaks form. Whisk about a quarter of the egg whites into tofu mixture in saucepan. Scrape tofu mixture over remaining egg whites and fold together just until combined. Spoon into the prepared soufflé dish.

4. Bake until puffy, set, and lightly browned on top, about 35 minutes. Serve immediately.

Make-Ahead Tip: Tofu mixture can be prepared up to a day ahead. Press plastic wrap against the surface of the mixture and refrigerate. Let stand at room temperature to let warm slightly before using.

Citrusy Green Tea Ice

Here's a novel way to serve green tea, which is touted as having all sorts of medicinal qualities, including anticancer benefits.

MAKES ABOUT TWELVE $\frac{1}{2}$-CUP SERVINGS
Prep: 10 minutes / Refrigerate: 2 hours, plus freezing time

8 tea bags green tea

$\frac{2}{3}$ cup organic sugar (evaporated cane juice)

$\frac{1}{4}$ cup honey

$1\frac{1}{2}$ cups orange juice

$\frac{1}{4}$ cup freshly squeezed lemon juice

2 teaspoons peeled, grated fresh ginger (optional)

1. In a medium-size saucepan, bring 2 cups water to a boil. Remove from heat, add tea bags, and let steep for 5 minutes. Remove tea bags, gently squeeze out liquid into pan, and discard bags. Stir in sugar until dissolved. Stir in honey until blended. Add orange juice, lemon juice, and ginger, if using. Cover and refrigerate for at least 2 hours, or until well chilled.

2. Freeze in an ice cream maker according to manufacturer's instructions. Or, to make in the refrigerator freezer, pour tea mixture into a 13 x 9 x 2-inch or an 8 x 8 x 2-inch metal baking pan. Place the pan in the freezer until solid around sides and just lightly slushy in center, about 3 hours. Break up frozen mixture around edges of pan. Spoon entire mixture into a food processor and process just until smooth. It should still be very slushy. Serve immediately as a frozen slush or scrape back into pan and freeze until solid. Let soften slightly before serving.

Make-Ahead Tip: Ice can be frozen for up to a month.

Pomegranate-Blueberry Ice

Both blueberries and pomegranates are rich in antioxidants, and this ice incorporates them into a purple, explosive-tasting dessert. Some research suggests that pomegranate juice may have anti–prostate cancer properties. The juice comes bottled and can be found in the health food, produce, or beverage section of your supermarket.

MAKES ABOUT TEN $\frac{1}{2}$-CUP SERVINGS
Prep: 15 minutes / Refrigerate: 2 hours, plus freezing time

  2 cups frozen blueberries
  $\frac{2}{3}$ cup organic sugar (evaporated cane juice)
  $\frac{1}{4}$ cup honey
  $\frac{1}{4}$ teaspoon ground cinnamon
  $\frac{1}{8}$ teaspoon ground cloves
  2 cups pomegranate juice
  2 tablespoons freshly squeezed lime juice

1. In a small saucepan, combine blueberries, 1 cup of water, sugar, honey, cinnamon, and cloves. Bring to a simmer over medium heat and cook for 2 minutes, stirring occasionally. Remove from heat and puree in a blender (place a towel over the lid to firmly hold it down). Strain mixture through a sieve into a medium-size bowl, pressing it through with the back of a spoon or with a rubber spatula. Discard any skins or other solids in sieve. Stir pomegranate juice and lime juice into blueberry mixture. Cover and refrigerate for at least 2 hours or until well chilled.

2. Freeze in an ice cream maker according to manufacturer's instructions. Or, to make in the refrigerator freezer, pour pomegranate mixture into a 13 x 9 x 2-inch or an 8 x 8 x 2-inch metal baking pan. Place in freezer until solid around sides of pan and just lightly slushy in center, about 3 hours. Spoon entire mixture into a food processor and process just until smooth but still very slushy. Serve immediately as a frozen slush or scrape back into the pan and freeze until solid. Let soften slightly before serving.

Make-Ahead Tip: Ice can be frozen for up to a month.

Dried Fruit and Pear Compote with Chai Tea

The secret to the flavor of this compote is chai tea, which comes in a green version and can be found in the coffee and tea section of your supermarket. Green tea is touted as possessing cancer-fighting properties. If the dried figs are not available, you can substitute prunes. The fennel seeds add an interesting flavor note.

Serving Suggestions: Spoon over soy vanilla ice cream or hot oatmeal, or serve on its own as a snack or dessert.

MAKES EIGHT $\frac{1}{2}$-CUP SERVINGS
Prep: 20 minutes / Cook: 20 minutes / Refrigerate: 3 hours or overnight

> 4 chai tea bags (green tea)
>
> $\frac{3}{4}$ cup (4 ounces) dried figs, stems removed and halved lengthwise, or prunes, halved lengthwise
>
> $\frac{3}{4}$ cup (4 ounces) dried apricots, halved lengthwise
>
> $\frac{1}{4}$ cup honey
>
> 2 tablespoons packed light or dark brown sugar
>
> $\frac{1}{4}$ teaspoon crushed fennel seeds
>
> 2 strips lemon zest (about $2\frac{1}{2}$ x $\frac{3}{4}$ inch)
>
> 2 firm ripe pears (about 1 pound), peeled, halved through stems, cored, and thinly sliced crosswise
>
> $\frac{1}{3}$ cup dried cranberries (optional)
>
> 1 tablespoon freshly squeezed lemon juice

1. In a medium-size saucepan, bring 2 cups of water to a boil. Remove from heat, add tea bags, and let steep 3 to 5 minutes. Remove tea bags, squeeze out liquid into pan, and discard bags. Add figs, apricots, honey, sugar, fennel seeds, and lemon zest. Bring to a gentle simmer, stirring to dissolve sugar, and simmer, covered, for 8 minutes.

2. Stir in pears and cranberries, if using. Press fruit down to submerge it in liquid. Return to simmer and cook, covered, until pears are just tender, about 8 minutes, depending on ripeness of pears. Remove from heat and stir in lemon juice. Pour into a bowl and set aside to cool. Refrigerate, covered, for at least 3 hours or overnight. Serve warm, cool, or at room temperature.

Make-Ahead Tip: Compote can be refrigerated for up to two weeks.

Individual Summer (and Winter) Puddings

These puddings are based on the British dessert made popular years ago in food magazines. Since this recipe relies on frozen fruit, the puddings can be made anytime, regardless of the season. Whole-wheat bread, with its extra bit of fiber and nutrients, replaces the usual refined white bread. And there's only 1 gram of fat per pudding.

MAKES 4 SERVINGS
Prep: 20 minutes / Cook: 2 minutes / Refrigerate: 6 hours or overnight

  1 package (16 ounces) frozen mixed berries (quarter strawberries if whole and large)
  $\frac{1}{4}$ cup plus 2 tablespoons packed light brown sugar
  $\frac{1}{4}$ cup seedless all-fruit raspberry jam or cherry preserves
  1 teaspoon grated lemon zest
  1 tablespoon freshly squeezed lemon juice
  2 tablespoons cassis or raspberry liqueur (optional)
  3 slices day-old whole-wheat bread (see Note), crusts removed and cut into
      $\frac{3}{4}$-inch cubes (about 2 cups)
  $\frac{3}{4}$ cup tofu vanilla ice cream (optional, for topping)

1. In a medium-size nonstick saucepan, combine berries, sugar, jam, and lemon zest. Bring to a simmer over medium-low heat and cook for 2 minutes. Remove from heat and stir in lemon juice and liqueur, if using. Set aside to cool.

2. Meanwhile, divide about half of bread cubes into the bottoms of four 1-cup dessert dishes. Spoon a total of $\frac{1}{4}$ cup of berry mixture over bread in each dish. Using the back of a spoon, lightly press mixture level.

3. Top with remaining bread cubes and remaining berry mixture, dividing equally. Cover with plastic and refrigerate for at least 6 hours or overnight.

4. If using ice cream, let stand until soft-serve consistency. Dollop over puddings, and serve.

Note: If bread is not stale, toast slices in a toaster at lowest setting until dry but not browned. Let cool and cut into $\frac{3}{4}$-inch cubes.

Make-Ahead Tip: Puddings can be refrigerated for up to two days.

Very Rich Chocolate Mousse

Everyone thinks this is the real thing, rich with heavy cream and eggs—silken tofu is the secret behind the smooth, creamy texture. The maple syrup adds sweetness and a depth of flavor. This mousse is definitely high in calories, but keep in mind there is no animal fat in this recipe. And some experts suggest that the stearic fatty acid in chocolate may impede the growth of prostate cancer cells.

Serving Suggestions: Let the mousse stand at room temperature for a short time and the texture will become more puddinglike. The softened mousse also can be used as a frosting for a cake—it's similar to a chocolate ganache, a rich mixture made with heavy cream.

MAKES EIGHT $\frac{1}{4}$-CUP SERVINGS
Prep: 10 minutes / Cook: 5 minutes / Refrigerate: 2 hours

  1 box (12.3 ounces) silken soft tofu

  2 teaspoons pure vanilla extract

  2 cups good-quality semisweet chocolate chips

  $\frac{1}{2}$ cup maple syrup

  1 teaspoon grated orange zest (optional)

1. In a small food processor, blend together tofu and vanilla until smooth.

2. In the top of a double boiler or in a metal bowl set over saucepan of simmering water, melt together chocolate and maple syrup, stirring occasionally. Let cool slightly.

3. Add chocolate mixture and optional orange zest to tofu in processor. Blend until smooth. Transfer to a bowl and refrigerate until thoroughly chilled, about 2 hours.

Make-Ahead Tip: Mousse can be refrigerated for up to three days.

Pumpkin Flan with Caramel Sauce

There are no egg yolks or saturated fat in this dessert, the usual hallmarks of most flans—silken tofu makes the flan creamy. Amazingly, a serving is only a little more than 100 calories, with only 1 gram of fat. To make individual flans, see below.

MAKES 10 SERVINGS
Prep: 15 minutes / Cook: 50 minutes / Refrigerate: 4 hours or overnight

$^2/_3$ cup organic sugar (evaporated cane juice)

1 cup unsweetened soy milk

$^3/_4$ cup canned pumpkin puree (not pie filling)

$^1/_2$ cup (4 ounces) silken tofu, drained and blotted dry with paper towels

$^1/_3$ cup honey

$^3/_4$ cup liquid egg substitute

1 teaspoon pure vanilla extract

$^3/_4$ teaspoon ground cinnamon

$^1/_2$ teaspoon ground ginger

$^1/_2$ teaspoon salt

1. Heat oven to 350°F. Set a 9-inch deep-dish pie plate (or an 8 x 8 x 2-inch square baking dish) into a roasting pan. Fill pan with hot water to come $^3/_4$ inch up side of pie plate.

2. Place sugar in a small, heavy-bottomed saucepan over medium heat and cook until melted and golden brown, stirring more frequently as sugar starts to melt and color, 3 to 5 minutes. Immediately pour into pie plate. Remove plate from water bath and quickly swirl melted sugar to coat bottom and partially up sides of dish. Return plate to water bath.

3. In a blender or small food processor, blend together soy milk, pumpkin, tofu, honey, egg substitute, vanilla, cinnamon, ginger, and salt until smooth. Pour into the pie plate.

4. Bake until a knife inserted near the center comes out clean, 45 to 50 minutes. Remove the baking dish from the water bath to a wire rack and let cool for 1 hour. Cover with plastic wrap and refrigerate for 4 hours or overnight.

5. To unmold, run a thin-bladed knife around the edge of the plate. Invert a serving plate over the pie plate, and turn both over together, shaking gently to release. Remove pie plate and scrape any remaining caramel onto flan. Cut into serving portions and serve.

Make-Ahead Tip: Flan can be refrigerated for up to two days.

Individual Flans: Set six 6-ounce custard cups in a 13 x 9 x 2-inch baking dish. Fill baking dish with hot water to come three-quarters up sides of custard cups. Caramelize the sugar as directed and divide among custard cups, swirling to coat bottom of each and partially up sides. Prepare custard as directed, divide equally among cups, and bake as directed.

Maple-Pecan Bread Pudding

There are no egg yolks or dairy in this dense bread pudding.

MAKES 8 SERVINGS

Prep: 20 minutes / Bake: 55 minutes

> Light olive oil, for baking dish
> 4 slices day-old whole-grain bread (see Note), cut into 1-inch cubes (about
> $3\frac{1}{2}$ cups)
> $1\frac{3}{4}$ cups unsweetened soy milk
> $\frac{1}{2}$ cup liquid egg substitute
> 2 teaspoons pure vanilla extract
> $\frac{3}{4}$ teaspoon ground cinnamon
> $\frac{1}{4}$ teaspoon ground nutmeg
> Pinch of salt
> $\frac{1}{3}$ cup maple syrup, plus additional for drizzling
> $\frac{1}{3}$ cup chopped pecans or Brazil nuts

1. Heat oven to 325°F. Coat an 8 x 8 x 2-inch square baking dish with oil.

2. Scatter bread cubes in an even layer in the prepared dish.

3. In a large bowl, whisk soy milk, egg substitute, vanilla, cinnamon, nutmeg, salt, and $\frac{1}{3}$ cup maple syrup until blended. Pour over bread, pressing down cubes. Sprinkle with nuts.

4. Bake until puffed and golden, 50 to 55 minutes—a knife inserted in center should come out clean. Cool on a wire rack at least 15 minutes. Serve warm, drizzling with maple syrup, if desired.

Note: If bread is not stale, toast slices in a toaster at lowest setting until dry but not browned. Cool and cut into cubes.

Make-Ahead Tip: Pudding can be refrigerated for two days and rewarmed in a 350°F oven or microwave.

Orange Cream Cheese Frosting

Smooth and creamy, this frosting easily spreads over the top of a cake and then drips down the sides. No dairy here—instead, soy cream cheese, and the brand I prefer for flavor is Tofutti. Keep in mind, it does contain partially hydrogenated soybean oil, so use it only from time to time.

Serving Suggestions: Spread over A Rich Carrot Bundt Cake (page 286), Spicy Gingerbread (page 296), or other plain cakes that need a little dressing up.

MAKES ABOUT 1 CUP
Prep: 5 minutes

1 container (8 ounces) nondairy imitation cream cheese (soy based)

1 cup organic sugar (evaporated cane juice)

2 tablespoons orange juice concentrate

$\frac{1}{8}$ teaspoon salt

In a food processor, process together all the ingredients just until smooth, about 10 seconds. Refrigerate until ready to use.

Make-Ahead Tip: Frosting can be refrigerated for up to two days.

Lemon Glaze

To add a special flavor interest to a plain cake such as carrot (page 286) or lemon poppy seed (page 276), spoon this warm glaze over a still-warm cake, with holes you've poked in the top so the glaze can soak in. To make an orange glaze, see the variation below.

Serving Suggestions: In addition to dressing up a cake, spoon a little over nondairy ice cream, cut-up fruit, or the top of a fresh fruit tart.

MAKES A SCANT $\frac{1}{2}$ CUP
Prep: 5 minutes / Cook: 1 minute

$\frac{1}{3}$ cup organic sugar (evaporated cane juice)
$\frac{1}{2}$ teaspoon grated lemon zest
$\frac{1}{4}$ cup freshly squeezed lemon juice

In a microwave-safe bowl, stir together all the ingredients. Microwave at full power until hot, stirring occasionally until sugar is dissolved, 45 to 50 seconds. (This can also be done in a small saucepan over medium-low heat.)

Make-Ahead Tip: Glaze can be refrigerated for up to a week and then gently reheated.

Orange Glaze: Substitute orange zest and juice for the lemon zest and juice.

Creamy Raspberry Sauce

Silken tofu is the secret ingredient. For a slightly less intense raspberry flavor, reduce the amount of berries from 1 cup to ½ cup. You can also substitute blueberries or strawberries.

Serving Suggestions: Spoon over a fruit sorbet or ice, a bowl of fresh fruit, a piece of lightly toasted low-fat pound cake, or any other dessert that could use a little saucing.

MAKES ABOUT 1 CUP

Prep: 5 minutes

> 1 cup (8 ounces) silken tofu, drained and blotted dry on paper towels
>
> 1 cup raspberries, blueberries, or strawberries, thawed if frozen
>
> 2 tablespoons confectioners' sugar
>
> 1 teaspoon pure vanilla extract
>
> ½ teaspoon freshly squeezed lemon juice

In a blender or food processor, puree together all the ingredients until silky smooth.

Make-Ahead Tip: Sauce can be refrigerated for up to two days.

Creamy Tofu Topping with Citrus

The addition of a little soy cream cheese makes this topping especially rich. You can vary the flavoring by adding 2 to 3 tablespoons of raspberry, strawberry, or whatever flavor jam you like—omit the coconut extract if you use the jam.

Serving Suggestions: Spoon over Individual Summer (and Winter) Puddings (page 308), a bowl of plain fruit, slices of Spicy Gingerbread (page 296), or Dried Fruit and Pear Compote with Chai Tea (page 307).

MAKES $\frac{2}{3}$ CUP
Prep: 10 minutes / Refrigerate: 1 hour

$\frac{1}{2}$ cup (4 ounces) silken tofu, drained and blotted dry with paper towels

3 tablespoons confectioners' sugar

2 tablespoons nondairy imitation cream cheese (soy based)

$\frac{1}{2}$ teaspoon freshly squeezed lime or lemon juice

1 teaspoon pure vanilla extract

3 drops coconut extract (optional)

Pinch grated nutmeg

In a small food processor, or in a tall glass and using a hand blender, blend together all the ingredients until smooth, about 1 minute. Scrape into a bowl and chill at least 1 hour.

Make-Ahead Tip: Topping can be refrigerated for up to three days.

Hot Chocolate Sauce

This tastes like the real thing, and actually it is! And no one would guess that tofu has been blended in to contribute a dose of isoflavones. Some even suggest that the stearic fatty acid in chocolate may impede the growth of prostate cancer cells

Serving Suggestions: Spoon over your favorite nondairy ice cream, over strawberries, or over a plain piece of cake.

MAKES ABOUT 1 CUP
Prep: 10 minutes / Cook: 3 minutes

> 1 ounce unsweetened chocolate, chopped
>
> 2 tablespoons unsweetened cocoa powder
>
> $\frac{1}{2}$ cup (4 ounces) silken tofu, drained and blotted dry with paper towels
>
> $\frac{1}{2}$ cup packed light brown sugar
>
> 3 tablespoons maple syrup
>
> 2 tablespoons unsweetened soy milk

1. In a blender, process together chocolate and cocoa powder until chocolate is finely ground, about 1 minute. Add tofu, sugar, maple syrup, and soy milk and blend until smooth.

2. Scrape into a small saucepan. Bring to a simmer over low heat and cook, stirring constantly, until chocolate is melted and sauce is smooth, about 3 minutes. Use sauce hot or warm.

Make-Ahead Tip: Sauce can be refrigerated for up to four days. Reheat it in a microwave, stirring every 15 seconds, until warmed. This can also be done in a small saucepan over low heat.

Macerated Strawberries

It takes just minutes to prepare this fruit topping. For a slightly richer flavor, add a splash of pure vanilla extract.

Serving Suggestions: Spoon over a small wedge of Hazelnut Sponge Cake (page 288), a square of Orange–Almond Snack Cake (page 294), an airy serving of Soufflé à l'Orange, (page 304) or a scoop or two of your favorite soy ice cream.

MAKES ABOUT 4 CUPS
Prep: 20 minutes

> 2 pints strawberries, hulled and quartered
> 3–5 tablespoons light brown sugar

In a medium-size bowl, toss together strawberries and sugar and let stand at least 15 minutes for sugar to dissolve.

Make-Ahead Tip: Berries can be made up to four hours ahead.

THOSE WHO HELPED

First there was my prostate cancer diagnosis, and then there was this book.

After my initial diagnosis of prostate cancer, Dr. Tom Reynolds, Susan McQuillan, Vicki Winter, Fred Maccaron, Dui Seid, Dora Jonassen, and Harry Ellsworth all helped me to sort through the initial decisions, and held my hand when I needed that.

And then there is Larry LaVigne II—his TLC as well as his own special brand of humor dispelled the dark moments. He also sampled a lot of the food in this book, and despite his strong dislike of any dish lacking meat or animal fat (that's his New Orleans background), he offered some very constructive critiques, in addition to his usual, "Dude! This dish needs meat!" His kitchen in Hartford became a home away from home when I needed a change of scenery.

Susan McQuillan, a good friend, a registered dietitian, and a collaborator with me on several cookbook projects, helped develop recipes, answered my nutrition questions, and performed an insightful edit on Chapter I, Prostate-Healthy Eating. Her daughter Molly, who celebrated her seventh birthday while I was writing this book, was part of my tasting panel, along with a couple of her friends. Molly also contributed several recipe ideas.

Other friends who sampled dishes and helped me to fine-tune the recipes were: Vicki Winter, Fred Maccaron, Dui Seid, Dora Jonassen (who has always provided a safe haven in New York City), Tom Votta, Harry Ellsworth, Stephen Frankel, Jimmy Staffer, and my ninety-something parents, Arthur and Gertrude, who were unexpectedly introduced to the wonders of tofu and pomegranate juice late in life.

Tom Critchley, a neighbor and friend, and also a fellow prostate cancer survivor, tasted some of my food, and our weekly luncheons at Fanizzi's restaurant in Provincetown, Massachusetts, became a forum for our respective prostate issues. Often conversations at surrounding tables seemed to stop as we discussed how our incontinences were lessening, as well as other pressing issues.

John Leo, as he has done in the past, approached my food with his own special culinary insights (often tempered by the mantra, "More kielbasa"), and I am the better man for it.

Other food professionals I've worked with over the years who developed recipes for this book are Sarah Reynolds, Donna Meadow, and Paul Piccuito, who made some great desserts. Stephen Frankel and Jimmy Staffer each contributed a recipe from their pasts.

Patty Santelli, a food and nutrition consultant who has worked with me on other projects, nutritionally analyzed every recipe in this cookbook so I could adjust them to achieve my goal of creating food that is generally low-calorie, high-fiber, and low in saturated fat.

Good friends Tom Reynolds and Rob Arnold allowed me take over the kitchen in their home in Rancho Mirage, California and were daring enough to let me prepare a practically all soy meal for some of their friends. The results? Everyone cleaned their plates.

Jane Dystel, my agent, enthusiastically supported the idea of a prostate cancer cookbook from the very beginning, and she, along with Miriam Goderich, at Dystel & Goderich Literary Management, helped me shape the initial book proposal.

And I always welcome the opportunity to work with Leslie Stoker at Stewart, Tabori & Chang, a civilized and gracious publisher and editor, in the best sense.

PROSTATE CANCER RESOURCES

American Cancer Society
(800) 277-2345
www.cancer.org
The organization provides information about cancer and support groups and funds research and community education.

American Foundation for Urologic Disease
(800) 828-7866
www.afud.org
The foundation provides information about urological conditions as well as prostate cancer, impotence, support networks, and clinical research.

American Institute for Cancer Research
(800) 843-8114
www.aicr.org
The cancer charity fosters research on diet and cancer prevention and educates the public about the results.

Cancer Care, Inc.
(800) 813-4673
www.cancercare.org
Founded in 1944, this national nonprofit organization provides free professional support services with trained oncology social workers to anyone affected by cancer—people with cancer, caregivers, children, loved ones, and the bereaved.

Cancer Research Institute
(800) 992-2623
www.cancerresearch.org
For five decades, the institute has been a sustaining force in cancer and immunology research.

Man to Man
(800) 227-2345
www.cancer.org, link to Man to Man
The American Cancer Society program helps men and their families cope with prostate cancer by providing community-based education and support to patients and their family members. Side by Side is a separate support group for wives and partners.

National Cancer Institute
(800) 422-6237
www.nci.nih.gov
An organization within the National Institutes of Health offering information about cancer treatments and clinical trials.

National Prostate Cancer Coalition
(888) 245-9455
www.pcacoalition.org
The coalition focuses on prostate cancer awareness, outreach, and advocacy.

Prostate Cancer Foundation
(800) 757-2873
www.prostatecancerfoundation.org
Formerly CapCure and founded by financier Michael Milken, the foundation is dedicated to finding better treatments and a cure for recurrent prostate cancer.

Prostate Cancer Research Institute (PCRI)
(800) 641-7274
www.prostate-cancer.org
The institute's mission is to educate patients and their families about prostate cancer and to support research.

Prostate Forum
(434) 974-1303
www.prostateforum.com
Dr. Charles (Snuffy) E. Myers, Jr., MD, a medical oncologist and prostate cancer survivor, heads a prostate cancer clinic near Charlottesville, Virginia, and lectures widely.

Prostate Pointers
www.prostatepointers.org
Web-based discussion and information about prostate cancer.

PSA Rising
www.psa-rising.com
The patient-centered news source and resource portal provides information about medical, scientific, and social aspects of prostate cancer survival.

US TOO
(800) 808-7866, support hot line
www.ustoo.com
This grassroots organization, started by prostate cancer survivors, provides information about prostate cancer and support groups.

BIBLIOGRAPHY

American Institute for Cancer Research. *The New American Plate Cookbook: Recipes for a Healthy Weight and a Healthy Life.* Berkeley: University of California Press, 2005.

Arnot, Dr. Bob. *The Prostate Cancer Protection Plan: The Foods, Supplements and Drugs That Could Save Your Life.* Boston: Little, Brown and Company, 2000.

Berley, Peter. *The Modern Vegetarian Kitchen.* New York: Regan Books, HarperCollins Publishers, 2000.

Bishop, Jack. *A Year in a Vegetarian Kitchen: Easy Seasonal Suppers for Family and Friends.* New York: Houghton Mifflin Company, 2004.

Blute, MD, Michael, Editor in Chief. *Mayo Clinic on Prostate Health.* Rochester, MN: Mayo Health Clinic Health Information, 2003.

Bostwick, MD, David G., et al. *American Cancer Society Prostate Cancer: What Every Man—and His Family—Needs to Know,* (rev.ed.). New York: Villard, 1999.

Brown, Sarah. *The Vegetarian Bible: The Complete Illustrated Guide to Vegetarian Food & Cooking.* Pleasantville, NY: Reader's Digest Association, 2002.

Criscuolo, Claire. *Claire's Corner Copia Cookbook: 225 Homestyle Vegetarian Recipes from Claire's Family to Yours.* New York: A Plume Book, Penguin Books, 1994.

Dorso, M. D., Michael A. *Seeds of Hope: A Physician's Personal Triumph Over Prostate Cancer.* Battle Creek, MI: Acorn Publishing, 2000.

Dragonwagon, Crescent. *Passionate Vegetarian.* New York: Workman Publishing, 2002.

Family Circle, Editors of, and David Ricketts. *The Family Circle Cookbook: New Tastes for New Times.* New York: Simon & Schuster, 1992.

Ginsberg, Beth, and Mike Milken. *The Taste for Living Cookbook: Mike Milken's Favorite Recipes for Fighting Cancer.* Santa Monica, CA: The Association for the Cure of Cancer of the Prostate (Cap CURE), 1998.

Golbitz, Peter. *Tofu & Soyfoods Cookery.* Sommertown, TN: Book Publishing Company, 1998.

Goldbeck, Nikki and David. *American Wholefoods Cuisine: Over 1300 Meatless, Wholesome Recipes from Short Order to Gourmet.* New York: A Plume Book, New American Library, 1983.

Jacobi, Dana. *Amazing Soy: A Complete Guide to Buying and Cooking This Nutritional Powerhouse, with 240 Recipes.* New York: William Morrow, 2001.

Kongpan, Sisamon. *The Best of Thai Vegetarian Food.* Bangkok: Sangdad Books, 2002.

Lange, MD, Paul H. *Prostate Cancer for Dummies,* New York: Wiley Publishing, Inc., 2003.

Lemlin, Jeanne. *Vegetarian Classics: 300 Essential and Easy Recipes for Every Meal.* New York: Quill, HarperCollins Publishers, 2001.

Leneman, Leah. *Vegan Cooking for Everyone: Over 250 Easy Recipes That Everyone Can Enjoy.* London: Thorson, HarperCollins, 2001.

MacNeil, Karen. *The Book of Whole Foods: Nutrition & Cuisine.* New York: Vintage Books, Random House, 1981.

Madison, Deborah. *This Can't Be Tofu! 75 Recipes to Cook Something You Never Thought You Would—and Love Every Bite.* New York: Broadway Books, 2000.

Marks, MD, Sheldon. *Prostate & Cancer: A Family Guide to Diagnosis, Treatment & Survival.* Fisher Books, 1999.

McEachern, Leslie. *The Angelica Home Kitchen: Recipes and Rabble Rousings from an Organic Vegan Restaurant.* Berkeley: Ten Speed Press, 2003.

Melina, MS, RD, Vesanto, and Brenda Davis, RD. *The New Becoming a Vegetarian: The Essential Guide to a Healthy Vegetarian Diet.* Sommertown, TN: Healthy Living Publications, 2003.

Moyad, MD, Mark A. *The ABC's of Nutrition and Supplements for Prostate Cancer.* Chelsea, MI: Sleeping Bear Press, 2000.

Myers, Jr., MD, Charles E., et al. *Eating Your Way to Better Health: The Prostate Forum Nutrition Guide.* Charlottesville, VA: Rivanna Health Publications, Inc., 2000.

Nasser, Christiane Dabdoub. *Classic Palestinian Cookery.* London: Saqi Book, 2001.

Oser, Marie. *More Soy Cooking: Healthful Renditions of Classic Traditional Meals.* New York: John Wiley & Sons, Inc., 2000.

Pirella, Chirstina. *Christina Cooks: Everything You Ever Wanted to Know About Whole Foods, But Were Afraid to Ask.* New York: HP Books, 2004.

Pratt, MD, Steven G., and Kathy Matthews. *Fourteen Foods That Will Change Your Life: Super Foods Rx.* New York: William Morrow, 2004.

Reader's Digest. *Vegetables for Vitality: 240 Delicious Recipes to Add Vegetables to Every Meal.* Pleasantville, NY: The Reader's Digest Association, Inc., 2004.

Ricketts, David. *Home Cooking Around the World: A Recipe Collection.* New York: Stewart, Tabori & Chang, 2001.

Ricketts, David, and Susan McQuillan. *Simply Healthful Pizzas and Calzones: Delicious New Low-Fat Recipes.* Shelbourne, VT: Chapters Publishing Ltd., 1994.

Ricketts, David, and Susan McQuillan. *Simply Healthful Fish: Delicious New Low-Fat Recipes.* Shelbourne, VT: Chapters Publishing Ltd., 1993.

Robertson, Laurel, et al. *The New Laurel's Kitchen: A Handbook for Vegetarian Cookery & Nutrition.* Berkeley: Ten Speed Press, 1986.

Robertson, Robin. *Vegan Planet: 400 Irresistible Recipes with Fantastic Flavors from Home and Around the World.* Boston: The Harvard Common Press, 2003.

Sanders, Buffy. *The Prostate Cancer Diet Cookbook: Cancer-Fighting Foods for a Healthy Prostate.* Gig Harbor, WA: Harbor Press, 2002.

Sandoval, Richard. *Modern Mexican Flavors: 125 Recipes from the Innovative Chef of Maya.* New York: Stewart, Tabori & Chang, 2002.

Sass, Lorna. *The New Vegan Cookbook: Innovative Vegetarian Recipes Free of Dairy, Eggs, and Cholesterol.* San Francisco: Chronicle Books, 2001.

Scardino, MD, Peter, and Judith Kelman. *Dr. Peter Scardino's Prostate Book: The Complete Guide to Overcoming Prostate Cancer, Prostatitis and BPH.* New York: Penguin, 2005.

Simon, MD, Harvey B. *The Harvard Medical School Guide to Men's Health: Lessons from the Harvard Men's Health Studies.* New York: Free Press, Simon & Schuster, Inc., 2002.

Strum, MD, Stephen B., and Donna Pogliano. *A Primer on Prostate Cancer: The Empowered Patient's Guide.* Hollywood, FL: The Life Extension Foundation, 2002.

Vegetarian Times, Editors of, and Lucy Moll. *Vegetarian Times Complete Cookbook.* New York: Wiley Publishing, Inc., 1995.

Walsh, MD, Patrick C., and Janet Farrar Worthington. *Dr. Patrick Walsh's Guide to Surviving Prostate Cancer.* New York: Warner Books, 2001.

Willet, MD, Dr. PH, Walter C. *Eat, Drink, and Be Healthy: The Harvard Medical School Guide to Healthy Eating.* New York: Free Press, Simon & Schuster, 2001.

CONVERSION CHARTS

WEIGHT EQUIVALENTS

The metric weights given in this chart are not exact equivalents, but have been rounded up or down slightly to make measuring easier.

Avoirdupois	Metric
$1/4$ oz	7 g
$1/2$ oz	15 g
1 oz	30 g
2 oz	60 g
3 oz	90 g
4 oz	115 g
5 oz	150 g
6 oz	175 g
7 oz	200 g
8 oz ($1/2$ lb)	225 g
9 oz	250 g
10 oz	300 g
11 oz	325 g
12 oz	350 g
13 oz	375 g
14 oz	400 g
15 oz	425 g
16 oz (1 lb)	450 g
$1^1/2$ lb	750 g
2 lb	900 g
$2^1/4$ lb	1 kg
3 lb	1.4 kg
4 lb	1.8 kg

VOLUME EQUIVALENTS

These are not exact equivalents for American cups and spoons, but have been rounded up or down slightly to make measuring easier.

American	Metric	Imperial
$1/4$ t	1.2 ml	
$1/2$ t	2.5 ml	
1 t	5.0 ml	
$1/2$ T ($1^1/2$ t)	7.5 ml	
1 T (3 t)	15 ml	
$1/4$ cup (4 T)	60 ml	2 fl oz
$1/3$ cup (5 T)	75 ml	$2^1/2$ fl oz
$1/2$ cup (8 T)	125 ml	4 fl oz
$2/3$ cup (10 T)	150 ml	5 fl oz
$3/4$ cup (12 T)	175 ml	6 fl oz
1 cup (16 T)	250 ml	8 fl oz
$1^1/4$ cups	300 ml	10 fl oz ($1/2$ pt)
$1^1/2$ cups	350 ml	12 fl oz
2 cups (1 pint)	500 ml	16 fl oz
$2^1/2$ cups	625 ml	20 fl oz (1 pint)
1 quart	1 liter	32 fl oz

OVEN TEMPERATURE EQUIVALENTS

Oven Mark	F	C	Gas
Very cool	250–275	130–140	$1/2$–1
Cool	300	150	2
Warm	325	170	3
Moderate	350	180	4
Moderately hot	375	190	5
	400	200	6
Hot	425	220	7
	450	230	8
Very hot	475	250	9

INDEX

shepherd's pie with sweet
potato topping, 182–83
turkey and bacon sandwich
with avocado-chipotle
mayonnaise, 85
see also Bacon, meatless soy;
Beef, ground, -style soy
protein; Frankfurters, soy;
Sausage links, soy
"Meatballs," herbed and
Parmesan, in tomato sauce, 178
in hero with mozzarella, 74
spaghetti with, 215
Mexican- and Tex-Mex-style
dishes:
black bean and tortilla casserole
with salsa, 154
black bean and vegetable
tostada with avocado and
lime, 83
black bean chili with chipotle,
155
breakfast burrito with red bell
pepper and zucchini, 273
chili con soy, 153
corn stew with red beans and
chiles, 104–5
quesadillas with tomatoes and
chiles, 62
rice and jack cheese casserole
with chiles and corn, 144
smoky cheese enchiladas, 171
Southwest lasagna with spinach
and pinto beans, 164–65
spinach enchiladas with jack
cheese and soybeans, 162–63
tomato salsa with serrano chile,
52
tortilla soup with serrano chile,
103
Milk, 19, 20
soy, 32, 35, 36–37
Modern Mexican Flavors
(Sandoval), 52
Modified citrus pectin (MCP),
29
Monkfish, roasted, with
tomatoes and spices, 210
Monounsaturated fat, 27, 30, 33

Monterey Jack-style soy cheese.
See Jack- or Monterey Jack-
style soy cheese
Moo shu, edamame, with
tortillas, 186–87
Moroccan spices, baked tuna
with honey glaze and, 190
Mousse, chocolate, very rich,
309
Mozzarella-style soy cheese, 36
broccoli rabe pizza with
tomato, 227
chicken Parmesan melt, 80
"meatball" hero with
mozzarella, 74
mushroom lasagna with red
bell pepper and edamame,
222–23
nutty lentil loaf with veggies
and mozzarella cheese,
158–59
pita pizzas with roasted
peppers, 67
roasted red pepper pizza, 226
sausage and mozzarella stuffed
bread, 86–87
tomato skillet pizza with
mozzarella and basil, 228
Muffins, banana spice, 282–83
Mushroom(s), 35
barley and edamame pilaf with
lemon and, 254
lasagna with red bell pepper
and edamame, 222–23
penne with gremolata and, 214
quinoa with red bell pepper
and, 149
shiitake, soy-glazed halibut
with, 207
and spinach manicotti, 224–25
three-, stroganoff with thyme,
179
tofu scramble with thyme and,
271
wild, barley risotto with
asparagus and, 145
wild, ragout, pumpkin polenta
with, 150–51
Mustard:

ginger dressing, 140
honey dressing, creamy, 135
-ketchup topping, 160–61
lemon sauce with horseradish,
257
lime salad dressing, 132
Mustard greens, 17, 30

N

Noodle(s):
soup with vegetables and
edamame, Thai, 98–99
see also Pasta
Nut(s), 30, 31, 34, 35
baked trail mix with dried
cranberries, 68
cranberry bread, 279
nutty lentil loaf with veggies
and mozzarella cheese,
158–59
nutty maple French toast, 272
and oat scones, 280–81
see also Brazil nut(s); Pecan(s)
Nutrition analysis, for recipes, 25

O

Oat(meal)(s), 31, 35
apple and pear crisp with
cranberries, 302
cookies with cranberries and
Brazil nuts, 301
and nut scones, 280–81
Obesity, 18, 19
Oils, 15, 30
olive, 30, 32, 33
Olive(s), 30
black, and sun-dried tomato
sauce, rigatoni with broccoli
and, 216
black, baked sea bass with
tomato and, 191
black, spread with sun-dried
tomatoes, 44
Olive oil, 30, 32, 33
Omega-3 essential fatty acids,
15, 18, 27, 33–34, 35, 189
Onion(s), 31
caramelized, crostini with red
wine and, 57